KICK MENST
IN THE NUTS

M000312278

By
T.C. Hale
& Two Other Guys

BIG FLIPPIN' DISCLAIMER

This book is not intended as a substitute for the medical recommendations of a physician or other healthcare provider. Don't be stupid. It's just a book. This book is intended to entertain and to offer information to help the reader cooperate with physicians and health professionals in a mutual quest of improved well-being.

The identities of people described in this book have been changed to protect confidentiality. Even when I talk about David Hasselhoff. That could be a totally different David Hasselhoff than the one you might be thinking of.

The Kick It in the Nuts series is written and published as an information resource and educational guide for both professionals and non-professionals. It should not be used to replace medical advice.

The publisher and the author are not responsible for any goods and/or services offered or referred to in this book and expressly disclaim all liability in connection with the fulfillment of orders for any such goods and/or services and for any damages, loss, or expense to person or property arising out of or relating to them. You are responsible for your own health and wellness.

PLEASE VISIT THE AUTHOR'S WEBSITE AT:

www.KickItInTheNuts.com

Or follow him on Twitter and Facebook:

www.twitter.com/KickItInTheNuts

www.facebook.com/KickItInTheNuts

ACKNOWLEDGEMENTS

Thank you to my co-authors and collaborators. Without your help and patience, this book would still be a big stack of ideas.

Special thanks to Sarah Griswold, for rewriting nearly every word of this book in the hopes of making me sound less stupid. It's fun to be able to say I wrote a book, even though meximelt and Fonzie are the only two words remaining from my original manuscript.

Thank you to my readers, editors and contributors: Sam Bangs, Alex and Red Donnally, Gabe Evans, Kinna McInroe, Elaine Alcala, Laura Hirsch and Monique Becker.

Thank you to my brother, Richard, who is also an author, for his insight into how to not be a sucky author. I don't understand why you haven't checked out his books yet. He writes great thrillers.

www.RichardCHaleAuthor.com

Finally, I'd like to thank you, the reader, for allowing me to entertain myself throughout this book, instead of just getting to the point, even though you may be experiencing cramps right now. I thank you for indulging me.

TABLE OF CONTENTS

KICK MENSTRUAL CRAMPS IN THE NUTS

Big Flippin' Disclaimer iii

Author's Website iv

Acknowledgements v

Introduction 1
  About The Authors 1

Chapter One 7
  Hi 7
  Why Am I Reading A Natural Health Book Written By A Comedian? 9
  About This Series Of Books 11
  Why Have I Never Heard This Information? 14
  How Medications Work 17
  Do I Qualify To Read This Book? 20
  How To Use This Knowledge 22
  Testing Tools You'll Need For This Book 25

Chapter Two 28
  What's With The Cramps? 28
  What Causes Cramps? 29
  Everything Goes Back To Digestion 30
  Why Am I Getting Cramps? My Friend Never Gets Cramps. 31
  All Cramps Are Not Created Equal 32
  Muscle Cramps And Calcium 33
  Calcium And The Overrated Vitamin D 34
  Why Did Blood Tests Tell Me I Had Low Vitamin D? 38
  Vitamin D And Heart Health 39
  Clinical Trials 41
  Calcium Following Sugar 43
  Joint Pain And Bone Spurs 45

Chapter Three   **47**

Blood Work, Body Chemistry And Imbalances   47

Blood Work And Working Symptomatically   47

Communicating With Your Doctor   50

Body Chemistry And Imbalances   52

"Let food be your medicine. Let medicine be your food."   54

The Argument That Changed The Course Of Medicine   54

Terrain Of The Body And Biochemical Individuality   56

Those Who Paved The Way   58

Intro To Imbalances   58

     Electrolyte Excess and Electrolyte Deficiency Imbalances   59

     Anabolic and Catabolic Imbalances   59

     Beta Oxidizer and Tricarb Oxidizer   59

     Sympathetic and Parasympathetic Imbalances   59

     Acid and Alkaline Imbalances   60

Chapter Four   **61**

Testing   61

Advanced Tests   66

Let's Get To Testing...   68

Data Tracking Sheet   70

The Coalition   71

Testing Procedures   73

     Frequently Used Tests   73

     Intermittent Tests   76

     Bonus Tests   82

Chapter Five   **86**

Understanding Your Imbalances   86

Understanding The Data   88

How Symptoms Can Help   89

Imbalance Guide   92

Sorting Out The Data   93

Imbalance Guide Content   94

     Symbols Key   94

     Electrolyte Status   94

     Circadian Rhythm (Cellular Permeability)   95

     Energy Production   97

     Autonomic Nervous System   98

     Acid/Alkaline Balance   99

Digestive Issues   99

Okay, I Can Add Check Marks... Now What?   100

What Is My Priority?   102

Understanding Fluctuations In Your Numbers   102

Low Potassium Issues   104

Be Patient   105

Using The Coalition   107

Optimal pHs According To Breath Rate   109

Calling In A Professional   109

Chapter Six   **111**

Imbalances   111

Imbalances And Your Symptoms   111

Electrolyte State   113

    Imbalance - Electrolyte Deficiency   113

    Imbalance - Electrolyte Excess   119

Cellular Permeability   121

    Imbalance - Anabolic   122

    Imbalance - Catabolic   124

Energy Production   126

    Imbalance - Tricarb Oxidizer   127

    Imbalance - Beta Oxidizer   128

Autonomic Nervous System   129

    Imbalance - Parasympathetic   130

    Imbalance - Sympathetic   131

pH Balance   131

    Imbalance - Tending to Alkalosis   133

    Imbalance - Tending to Acidosis   135

Chapter Seven   **137**

Digestion   137

Losing Your Period And Pre-Menopausal Symptoms   138

Sex Is The Blossom Of Life   140

How Digestion Works   142

More On HCL   144

Minerals And HCL   146

H. Pylori   147

Chapter Eight   **149**

Digestion Gone Wild   149

Reflux, Heartburn And GERD 149

Crohns, Colitis, And IBS 151

Let's Talk Crap 152

Burping, Bloating And Passing Gas 154

Digestive Enzymes 155

Conquering Our Food - Food Allergies 156

Birth Control Medications 159

Gallbladder Removal/Gallstones/Olive Oil-Lemon Drink 161

Liver Function 164

Chapter Nine **167**

Other Factors With Cramps 167

Chocolate, etc. 167

Cravings - Part Two 170

L.A.'s Finest 172

Sugars And Complex Carbs 174

What Carbs Should I Eat? 175

Hypoglycemics And Low Blood Sugar 176

Mining Your Own Body 177

Resilience Of The Body 178

Stress 180

Sun Exposure 182

Sea Salt 183

Bonus Insight 184

Chapter Ten **185**

Foods That Can Help 185

Diet Is Determined By Strength Of Digestion 189

Contradictions From Imbalance To Imbalance 189

Imbalance - Electrolyte Deficiency 190

Imbalance - Electrolyte Excess 193

Imbalance - Anabolic 195

Imbalance - Catabolic 197

Imbalance - Tricarb Fast Oxidizer (Carb Burner) 199

Imbalance - Beta Slow Oxidizer (Fat Burner) 200

Imbalance - Parasympathetic 201

Imbalance - Sympathetic 202

Imbalance - Tending To Acidosis 202

Imbalance - Tending To Alkalosis 204

Chapter Eleven   205

Using Supplements   205
What If I Hate Taking Supplements?   208
Where To Find It   209
What To Look For   210
Di-Calcium Phosphate   211
Magnesium Stearate   211
Gelatin vs. Vegetable Capsules   211
Whole Food/Complete Food Supplements   212
Vitamin C   214
When To Take Supplements   215
Vitamins   216
Minerals   216
Amino Acids   216
Digestive Enzymes   217
Probiotics   217

Chapter Twelve   219

Digestive Supplements   219
Hydrochloric Acid (HCL) Warning   220
HCL Protocol   220
What If I Don't Feel A Warming Sensation?   222
What If I Take Too Much?   223
What If My Stool Becomes Too Loose?   223
What If I Feel Heartburn?   224
Eating Carbs When You First Start Using HCL   226
H. Pylori   228
HCL With A Catabolic Imbalance   235
Bile Flow   237
What If My Gallbladder Was Yanked?   240
Digestive Enzymes   241
Sea Salt (Unrefined Salt)   243

Chapter Thirteen   245

Supplements For Specific Imbalances   245
Imbalance - Electrolyte Deficiency   248
Imbalance - Electrolyte Excess   249
Imbalance - Anabolic   250
Imbalance - Catabolic   251
Imbalance - Tricarb Fast Oxidizer (Carb Burner)   252

Imbalance - Beta Slow Oxidizer (Fat Burner)   252
Imbalance - Parasympathetic   253
Imbalance - Sympathetic   254
Imbalance - Tending To Acidosis   255
Imbalance - Tending To Alkalosis   255
Finding A Qualified Health Coach In Your Area   255

Chapter Fourteen   **257**
A Healthy Body In An Unhealthy World   257
Water   259
Shower Filters   261
Microwaves   262
What Am I Cooking In?   264
What's In My Mouth?   264
Smoking   264
Soda   265
Artificial Sweeteners   267
Antibiotics   268
Flu Shots   269
Alkalizing Water And Water Filters   269
What About Meat?   271
Vegan / Vegetarian   274
Organic vs. Conventional   277
Soil And Minerals   281

Chapter Fifteen (The Sum Up)   **284**
Review & Make Your Plan   284
Now What?   284
Bring It All Together   284
Fix Digestive Issues   286
Correct Your Imbalances   286
Monitor Your Numbers   287
Don't Work Against Yourself   287
Watch The Signs   288
Make Your Plan   289
Avoid Screwing Yourself Over   290
Finding Supplements   293
Continue To Learn   293
Hidden Chapter   293
Ask F'in Tony & The Community Forum   294

Book Updates   294
Follow Me   295
My First Movie   295
Your Top Secret Book Reader Code   295
Be Excited   295
Final Words   295

Appendix A   **296**
11-Parameter Urine Dipstick & Advanced Testing Details   296
11-Parameter Urine Dipstick   296
Advanced Tests   300
Tests You Can Do Now   300
Tests That Need Advanced Equipment And Education   304

Appendix B   **308**
Those Who Paved the Way   308
Dr. Carey Reams   308
Dr. Emanuel Revici   308
Thomas Riddick   309
Dr. Melvin Page   310
Recommended Reading   311

More About Tony   **312**

INTRODUCTION

About The Authors

Geez. Where do I start? My name is Tony Hale. I just use the pen name "T.C. Hale" because if you Google "Tony Hale" you find four hundred thousand pictures of Buster Bluth from *Arrested Development*. If you're unfamiliar with the actor, one of his first big national spots was that Volkswagen commercial with the guy doing the robot in his car. I can remember studying at The Groundlings when a girl in my class told me that her friend's name was Tony Hale too, and that he was the guy in the Volkswagen commercial. I recall thinking, "That bastard's going to call dibs on my name before I do," and that's pretty much how it's worked out. I run into Tony around town from time to time and he's actually a super nice guy. The first time a I met him, he was shopping at Whole Foods. I walked up to him, didn't say a word, and just handed him my driver's license. "No way!" he said after seeing my name.

Turns out, he was excited to meet me because he had heard of my existence since I have an acting credit that is listed on his IMDb.com page. When I was touring as a comic, I was dating a girl who booked one of the leads in an independent film called *Raging Hormones*. Visiting her on set, the director asked me to drive by in a scene and make fun of the main character. It earned me a film credit, but they attached it to the wrong Tony Hale. Since this was literally THE worst movie that has ever been created, I decided to let Tony keep the credit. Tony told me that he always wondered if that was a real movie and how it got on his resume. I let him know that he should be proud to have been involved in a film that was even more brilliant than *Gigli*. But, enough about my name already. What about the rest? How the hell did I get here?

I guess like most natural health and nutrition researchers, my background comes from a professional career in stand-up comedy. I found that, as I traveled across the country from city-to-city, if I had a show that didn't go well, I figured that town must be constipated. With the realization that very few things are ever funny when you can't poop, I began using science in my comedy career. Handing out laxatives at my show seemed odd at first... Um, I think that's as far as I can BS my way through that story. That's really not how it happened at all and I apologize for lying so early in our relationship. The truth is, yes, I toured as a comic, but the only thing I learned about natural health on the road was that, in the towns where people drank a lot of alcohol, their bodies were a lot fatter and I was a lot funnier.

I actually became a natural health and nutrition researcher by necessity. On Valentine's Day, 2003, I took my girlfriend at the time to see The Dan Band at the club, Hollywood and Highland. We had some of our friends meet us at the nightclub after the show. Most of the night, I talked over the loud music. The next day, my voice was gone and it never came back. Over the next year or so, 23 doctors, specialists, and surgeons couldn't figure out what the problem was. With each doctor and each medication, my health seemed to decline a little more. After exhausting my way through doctors, speech therapists, natural practitioners, and a six-figure accumulation of expenses, I told everybody to piss off and decided I was going to figure this out myself.

And that's what I did. Over the next six years I did nothing but read books, research nutrition experts, and attend workshops and seminars across the country. As I searched for my own answers, I kept stumbling across answers to problems that my friends were dealing with. I was so amazed to find explanations that I had never heard of that I started to share them with my friends. When I emailed my buddy Greg and explained to him some of the underlying issues that can make a person have to sit on the toilet twelve times a day, he ran some measurements on himself to see what the likely causes were and his chemistry matched up perfectly with most people who have similar issues. He tried the things I showed him and he was able to poop like a normal human, once or twice a day, instead of shooting soup out the back door all day.

As one friend would tell another friend, people kept emailing me and asking if I could help them understand their health issues. But I was working as a personal trainer and didn't have time to teach all those people how to look at their own chemistry to understand why they're dealing with what they're dealing with. That is, until a guy named Jim, who was so impressed with how I taught his friend how to understand and improve his own insomnia, offered me $500 to help him, too. That's when I realized, "Oh, this is a business." After all, I would have gladly paid someone $10,000 to help me correct my issues six years earlier. That's a lot of money, but it still would have saved me $90,000. With this revelation, I started a career as a health coach. I've never advertised, but today I help some of the biggest stars and most influential people in the entertainment industry better understand how they can use nutrition to improve their health. That is also what I'm going to do with you in these pages. Isn't that nice of me? You don't even have your own show and I'm still going to help you.

Before you look at anything I have to say as gospel, I want to make sure that I am very clear on the fact that I am not a doctor and I don't claim to be any sort of doctor or licensed professional. I don't even watch *House*. I used to think M*A*S*H was funny, but that hardly makes me a doctor. What I am is a guy who became fed up with the system and decided I would find my answers elsewhere. I'm just a guy who had no choice but to keep digging until solutions were uncovered. I had no choice because it was becoming clear that I wasn't going to be able to talk again unless I found some real answers. If it were anything else, I probably would have given up after two years. For example, if I were just walking with a limp, or I couldn't talk without whistling and spitting on people, or whatever the case may be, I probably would have just learned to live with it. But since I was very determined to get my voice back, I was willing to do the work. Remember, a stand-up comic with no voice is just a mime—and who wants to get punched in the face while they're working every day? You may not know this, but it has been statistically proven that 83% of the population would rather punch a mime than watch him try to entertain a crowd. Since I was so determined not to become another "mime statistic," you now get to reap the rewards of my years of research.

So, if you're looking for credentials, buy another book. I encountered plenty of professionals with credentials, certifications, licenses, awards, accolades, expensive offices... you name it. One guy even had a live ostrich that lived in the back yard of his office complex. (That didn't help, either.) The professionals I consulted had it all. Yet, none of them could help me. As a result of that experience, I find that I'm more interested in the truth than I am in credentials. Over the last 60 years, doctor after doctor who went outside the box to try to truly help patients (by working to correct the actual causes of their illness instead of just treating symptoms) have been stripped of their licenses, discredited, and basically run out of town. Sadly, this happens frequently. Seems like every time someone makes a significant splash in the mainstream market with any advances that could help people correct health issues naturally, that individual is discredited so that the masses will go back to spending billions on drugs that only mask their symptoms.

With these books, since my co-authors and I know this information will spread fast, we're going to go another route.

After all, when people finally get answers to problems they have been dealing with for decades, they talk about it. So we're setting up a system where people can learn about their body without having that system discredited. It can't be discredited because I am the voice and I'm telling you right now, I HAVE NO CREDENTIALS. I'm just a schmuck comedian and personal trainer who was willing to dig for some answers. And now I'm just sharing what I've learned with you, so you can dig for your answers a little quicker. Am I a doctor? No. Do I have a license? Heck no. Do we really need one more person following the same system that isn't working? I don't even shave every day, I've filed for bankruptcy in my life, I don't understand what color shirt I'm allowed to wear with brown pants, and I'm writing this book in my boxers. If you want to dig into my life, personally, you'll see that most of my clients call me "F#ckin' Tony" and I'm pretty sure they mean it. (When their friends ask, "Why can't you walk today?" My clients always reply, "F#ckin' Tony.") Honestly, a few clients decided that was my name and it just caught on. I realized the horrible reputation I must have when I walked into a birthday party for one of my clients last year. When my client announced to the room, "Everyone, this is Tony," thirty people I had never met simultaneously yelled, "F#ckin' Tony!!" Is that what you call somebody who has credentials?

Though I am not the only author in this series of books, I have been elected to be the voice and will be the only known author for many of our titles. In this book, as well as others in this series, my co-authors and contributors are made up of doctors, M.D.s, medical and natural health researchers, and some of the most well respected educators who teach doctors from all over the world about nutrition. When I traveled the country looking for answers, I found some individuals who have dedicated their lives to this work. I've approached many of them to help me in this effort. Though some have chosen to have their names added as co-authors to some of our titles, many are keeping their identity anonymous, so as to protect their practice and keep the powers-that-be from trying to discredit the amazing work they are doing.

Although I won't be sharing the names of most of my co-authors with you, I will share the pioneers from the 1930s and 1940s who first discovered these truths. That was the one constant that I seemed to find no matter who I talked to. Most of the experts I found had studied doctors from the 30s, 40s and 50s, back when a doctor was allowed to think. I'll talk about these pioneers throughout our time together, and I'll even point you in the direction of some of their amazing books so you can dig deeper if you find this information as interesting as I did.

Odds are someone who experienced incredible results recommended this book to you. So, my suggestion is for you to put your trust in the experience of your friend instead of the authorities that seem to be more interested in profit than results. After all, wasn't it Benjamin Franklin who once said, "Though I have welcomed the words from authorities my whole life, it might be time for them to go flog themselves," or something like that?

CHAPTER ONE

Hi

What's the one thing that could bring peace to the planet more than any other factor? What could bring more joy, alleviate more pain and reduce utter fear for every man and child in the world? Obviously the answer is... fewer menstrual cramps. How unfair is it that, every month, so many women have their lives turned upside-down by the tragic discomfort that is "Menstrual Cramps"? Why do so many women who are normally sweet and kind go through a transformation that makes the girls on *Flavor of Love* seem like Girl Scouts? Why must some women lie on their couches moaning "mommy help me" for two days when their period shows up, while others never experience any discomfort whatsoever?

There are actual reasons why, for some women, cramps are so severe, while others don't have to dread their period at all. Women all over the world are learning how they can look at their own body chemistry and physiology, and understand nutritional and lifestyle changes they can make to alleviate the horror they experience every month. And they're doing it without the help of medications.

If you're having an issue with menstrual cramps, or even if you've lost your period altogether, my co-authors and I will help you understand some of the actual causes behind your troubles and teach you how other women have been correcting them for years. Since it is widely accepted that so many women experience very difficult cramps, and that's just the way it is, I find that my clients are always surprised when they can find answers to questions like:

- Why do I get cramps, but my friend never does?
- If women can correct their cramps naturally, why has my doctor never shared this information?
- What is the actual cause behind my cramps?
- Why are some periods so much worse than others?
- How can I look at my own body chemistry and physiology to better understand the cause behind my cramps?
- What nutritional changes can help improve my cramps?
- Why does one remedy help my friend's cramps, but does nothing for me?

My co-authors and I agree that, for the most part, these questions haven't been addressed by traditional or alternative medicine. Even in the world of natural health, when someone provides a remedy for cramps, it's a one-size-fits-all approach. No one is looking at the individual, everyone is only looking at symptoms. Do shoes come only in one size? How about bras or even contact lenses? No. We look at people as individuals for just about anything they need, except their health. In the world of health care, we're a one-trick pony. We're like a 7-11 that sells only Zagnut bars. We look only at the symptoms instead of looking at the person who is suffering from the symptoms. And when our great, great, grandkids learn about our health care system in their history class, they will laugh at us. They will point, and they will laugh... and our only excuse will be that the characters on *Grey's Anatomy* were so dreamy, we just believed everything they said.

Kick Menstrual Cramps in the Nuts was written to help women look at their own biological identity, understand how their specific body is operating, and make the necessary changes to help their body function in a more optimal way... so they won't have to lie in bed for two days because they can't move without cussing at their husbands.

You and other readers, will learn how you can pick up inexpensive tools at just about any health food store and/or drug store, and run simple tests to investigate what may be the underlying cause behind the cramps you deal with every month. You will learn about imbalances in your body chemistry, how to understand the meaning of the imbalances, and even methods to improve those imbalances. You will find the simple charts and tools easy to use and helpful in monitoring your progress. This way, you can see if your body chemistry is moving toward a balanced state, even before your period shows up.

Best of all, this information will come to you from the point of view of a professional comedian who was forced into learning about nutrition and how the body really works because a long string of doctors couldn't help him. Hopefully, not only will you be entertained while you are being educated, you will learn from a regular person just like yourself—someone who speaks human English and doesn't hide the facts in medical terms that only six people on Earth can understand. The best part will be that the things you learn will actually make sense. Be excited! The answers you receive in this book will be more thrilling than your first "My Little Pony" charm bracelet.

Why Am I Reading A Natural Health Book Written By A Comedian?

While working at a seafood restaurant as a teenager, I once found a nickel inside a raw oyster. A nickel! It was as if the oyster was saving up to buy a pearl because nobody told him he was supposed to make his own. Well, in the same way that you can find something beautiful—like a pearl—in something so gross and snot-looking—like an oyster—you can also find something unexpected—like a nickel. My point is, I was surprised to find cash inside an oyster, but I was still able to use the cash on my way home that night when I stopped by the Taco Bell drive-through. So, just because you find some information on natural health in a place you might not expect, that doesn't mean it can't be useful to you. My nickel helped pay for a meximelt with no pico sauce, which was very useful to me. Even if the "nickel" you discover from this comedian is not useful to you, you can still drive through Taco Bell and say, "I was told that if I mentioned the book, *Kick Menstrual Cramps in the Nuts*, I would get a 50% discount." It won't reduce the cost of your meal, but I really like people talking about my books.

You may also be thinking, "Why am I reading a book about menstrual cramps that was written by someone who doesn't even have a uterus? I would have to kick *you* in the nuts for you to even understand where I'm coming from with my cramps." Yes, it is true that I am quite deficient in the category of "owning a uterus." However, since I had my own health issues that were plaguing me, I was forced to do a tremendous amount of research on my own. Sometimes when you're digging for gold, you come across a huge pile of silver. Even though I was only interested in "gold," I did realize that I had a lot of female friends who would be thrilled to learn about this "silver," so I began to share that knowledge with others. Once you get right down to it, it's all just science and that's what I'm going to explain in this book: The science behind the issues that may be plaguing you. If you're anything like other women with whom I have shared this information, reading this book could turn out to be even more spine-tingling than when you found out Joanie loved Chachi.

It is true that I have come across a bucket of knowledge that I am sharing with you, but I am still a comedian at heart and I have a hard time just spewing off science without having a little fun in the process. I normally amuse myself by making fun of those I shouldn't, presenting information in an inappropriate manner, or offending my readers for little to no reason at all. With that in mind, if you get offended easily, don't read this book. I have

10

another series called *Done With That* which can provide the same information in a less entertaining way. I promise I'll be a good little boy and on my best behavior in that series. I wrote that additional series so, if people sent me emails ranting about how I offended them, I could just reply stating, "Thank you for your input but the time has come for you to remember that I told you in the beginning to read *Done With Menstrual Cramps* instead if *Little House on the Prairie* is considered a risqué show in your house. Thank you for your continued support." Obviously, I have provided fair warning, don't you think? I can't wait to find out if you keep reading or not.

About This Series Of Books

In the *Kick It in the Nuts* series of natural health books, we'll be looking at our health, bodies, and nutrition in a way that is different from any other natural health book you've ever read. Instead of just looking at a condition and talking about all the "natural remedies" that have been known to work for that condition, we're going to spend most of our time looking at YOU - the individual. Focusing only on the condition or symptoms is the biggest mistake in the world of health. With this series of books, it is our goal to offer you other options.

Whether we're talking about the medical world, "alternative health" world, natural health or even nutrition—everyone seems to be making the same screw-up. They just look at a person's symptoms or condition instead of looking at the person who is dealing with the symptoms or condition. The ignorance behind this line of thinking is that just about every symptom or condition can have three or four different underlying causes. That's why so many "remedies" or methods will work great for one person with a particular symptom, but will make another person with that same symptom much worse. Nobody is looking at each individual and the actual cause of that symptom for *that* individual.

Well, I think this has gone on long enough. I understand how a person, and even a society, can get stuck believing one thing for years, or even decades, but there has to be a breaking point when reality sets in. Take *Baywatch*, for example. Television viewers made this program one of the top shows for nearly a decade. *The Guinness Book of World Records* had listed it as the most watched show of all time, while it was airing, with 1.1 billion viewers per week. So, we accepted that form of entertainment into our lives for a long, long time. But don't we feel much better now that we've realized the whole show was basically just half-naked ignorance with a drowning scene in the middle of each episode? Once we figured out why Pamela Anderson floated so well, and came to the realization that David Hasselhoff actually had a beer belly and had to suck in his gut for every beach scene, we decided it was time to see what else was on. And we all feel much better for the change. That's the type of relief you should be looking to gain through this series of books. I'll provide a new perspective that will help you unravel the benefits of looking at an individual's chemistry rather than just trying to treat a symptom or condition. I'm not saying that one point of view about health is right or wrong; my co-authors and I are just giving everyone an opportunity to see "what else is on."

I placed a disclaimer at the beginning of this book stating that this information should not replace any medical advice, etc., etc. Let's look a little deeper into this topic so you can have an understanding of what you might get out of this book. I don't want you to look at this book like it's going to be a tool to "beat my cramps." It's never a good idea to focus on trying to eliminate, declare war on, cure, or kick any problem in the nuts. The title to this series of books was just too funny not to use. But once you see the direction this knowledge can take you, you will see that trying to "beat" something is very rarely successful. Instead, the goal here will be to teach you about the body's operational systems and what imbalances might be moving in the wrong direction when common symptoms show up. You will also be taught how to look at your own chemistry and compare the issues you're having to what other people see when their chemistry is moving in a similar direction. Then I'm going to show you steps that others have taken in order to move their bodies back to a more balanced operational state. If you understand this objective, you will see that the goal should be to move toward health instead of trying to escape from, or beat down, symptoms or "disease." If an individual has good health, disease can't exist because that doesn't fit within the definition of health. Good health and disease can't coexist. By putting your attention on creating health, the body can often take care of problems on its own. That's how the body is intended to work.

Look at it this way... if you're in a dark, locked closet, there is nothing but darkness. You can't destroy the darkness. You can't beat it down or even run from it. To put your effort into changing that darkness into something else would be very frustrating and time consuming and your friends would say, "Hey, you've been in that closet for a long time... what the hell are you doing in there?" But if you turn on a light, the darkness will disappear on its own. It can't exist in a place where there is light. You didn't have to do anything to convince the darkness to leave or to stop tormenting you, you just invited something else into the closet that made it impossible for the darkness to exist there. You invited in the light and the darkness went away on its own.

By gaining the knowledge of how most healthy bodies seem to function, and how to look at your own body and find the systems that may not be running optimally, you will have the opportunity and the information to try to move yourself closer to health. In my experience, when I see people begin to work *with* their bodies instead of against them, many of the symptoms or issues that they are dealing with seem to improve—or disappear altogether. Of course, every person is different. There is no way to know what will happen with you. But if you had the knowledge to move yourself closer to health, wouldn't you want to take steps to implement that knowledge?

If you have ever read any of my other *Kick It in the Nuts* titles, or even my *Done With That* books, some content of this book may sound familiar to you. Much of this book will teach you how to look at you and your chemistry. Knowing your own chemistry is the most important factor when dealing with any health issue. In each title, I have given readers a foundation of information about chemical imbalances in the body, how to test their own chemistry, and how to view the information they find through testing. Those tools and methods never change no matter what health issue you would like to see improve. If you already have a good understanding of those techniques from one of my other books, you'll be miles ahead and you will be able to use this title to better understand how specific imbalances can relate to menstrual cramps. If you have friends who are suffering from a symptom discussed in one of my other books, you can feel confident recommending that book to them, even if you haven't read it. Because the same foundational principles covered here are covered in every one of the *Kick It in the Nuts* titles, your friends will understand common underlying causes to their issues in the same way you will, once you finish this book.

Why Have I Never Heard This Information?

Let's get started by putting down a foundation. That foundation is to answer the questions that will run through your head for the duration of this book. "Why have I never heard this stuff? Why didn't my doctor tell me this when I told him that my cramps are so bad that I can't even get out of bed? I even told my doctor what was coming out of my mouth last week when I was yelling at my husband for no reason! Is nothing in this book true or does my doctor hate me?"

While digging for answers, there was one topic that really changed the way I looked at my health, the choices I was making, and where I wanted to find help. Before I explain this, I just want to be clear that in no way am I saying that the entire medical world is a crapshoot, or that the entire system is more evil than that blonde guy from *The Karate Kid*. The advances and information that medical professionals and researchers have provided are truly amazing and many of them do indeed save and/or prolong lives. Even some medications that result in horrible side effects still provide you with the ability to buy yourself some time and fight off a certain death long enough to really improve your health or correct the underlying problem. The only knock on how the whole system works that I will cover here is this: We are given only half the story.

If you go out of town and I watch your dog while you're gone, then I'm a pretty nice guy. If you come home and there are no little piles of dog poop in your yard because I scooped it all up, then I'm an even nicer guy. Going above the call of duty, really. (Or the call of doodie depending on what we're talking about. [It makes me sad that I left that joke in here.]) You might be so appreciative that you take me to dinner and even buy me a hammock just because I always wanted one. But if every day while you were out of town I took the dog crap out of your yard and dumped it into the trunk of your car, then maybe I didn't tell you the whole story. Maybe you'll be less appreciative when you go to change a flat on the freeway. Sure I seemed like a nice guy, but I was leaving out some key information. Sometimes it's just nice to get the whole story, especially when we're talking about your life and your health.

With that in mind, here's the piece of information I came across again and again while I was trying to figure out why each doctor and each medication was making me worse instead of better. This is the piece of information that woke me up to the realization that it was time to put my health back into my own hands. Not that I didn't still need help from health professionals, but that I would become a player in the process of understanding what my options really were and what would be best for me. Here it is: *The vast majority of curricula that are taught in medical schools in this country were put together by organizations that were founded by, or are funded by, pharmaceutical companies.* Read that again.

15

So let me get this straight... The people who make the most money from our being sick are the same people who are teaching our doctors how to make us "healthy"? I need you to stop and think about that for just a second with the intelligent part of your brain—not the part that just listens to what we're taught or what the media or our friends say and just accepts it. You know what I mean. We've all been there. For years I thought it was cool to watch *The Dukes of Hazzard* because all my friends did, but I just had this hunch that maybe it was a pile of stupidity based around a girl with really small shorts.

My point is, think about that statement. How can that possibly be a piece of information that we accept as "just the way it is"? Pharmaceutical companies have total power to influence what our doctors are learning? When you're twelve years old, it's acceptable to watch Bo and Luke get into yet another car chase, but how long do we have to watch pharmaceutical sales rise, and illness and disease rise right along with it, before we demand a more intelligent system and more intelligent shows to watch? I mean, *America's Next Top Model*? Are we really progressing on either front?

By the way, if you happen to be having cramps right this minute, you'd probably love to punch me in the neck because I'm spending more time making jokes than I am explaining your issue. But if you read this whole book, and implement what is laid out in the pages to follow, I have a feeling I might turn out to be your new favorite person. All I'm saying is that if your cramps were to be eliminated or greatly reduced, it would probably change many aspects of your life. I have had girls ask me if they can buy me a pony or something to show their gratitude once they understood this information. (I no longer accept ponies due to a new city ordinance that was put in place to appease my neighbors. I do, however, accept gift cards from Apple or Whole Foods, and painted portraits of Ed Begley Jr.)

How Medications Work

Before we talk about how medications work, please make sure you understand that in no way am I suggesting you stop taking any medications you are currently using. In most cases, medication is doing a job, and the person taking it needs that medication to continue doing its job, so just chucking it in the trash could be dangerous for some people. But once you begin to understand why you're likely dealing with the issues that you're dealing with, and how some people improve them by making better choices and moving body chemistry in the right direction, then you can decide for yourself if you want to accomplish that. Once you improve some issues by making more ideal decisions, you can then discuss with your doctor the possibility of reducing, or removing, the need for any meds. But promise me you won't try to do this on your own because that's just dumb. If you're currently on any meds, chances are great that you are going to need some help from a professional, and the knowledge you receive in this book will be a great starting point to help you better choose and communicate with that professional. We'll talk about that more in chapter three under *Communicating with Your Doctor and Working with a Natural Practitioner.*

Here's how most drugs work. Nearly all drugs are synthetic, man-made substances; otherwise the manufacturer couldn't patent the drugs and make billions because it's not legal to patent a natural substance. However, most synthetic substances that enter the body will be filtered out by the liver and removed. That's the liver's job. So, if you put a drug in, the liver will filter it out and the drug won't be able to stay in the body and fulfill its purpose, rendering it worthless. To correct this, manufacturers upped the dosages in drugs to overwhelm the liver so enough of the drug can stay in your system and do the job (or give a physiological reaction) as it is intended to do. Well guess what? It works. The liver can't remove all of it and the drug often corrects the symptom it was intended to correct. Yet it does so at the cost of punching your liver in the mouth with every dose. Not only can this eventually lead to liver damage (which is why nearly every drug commercial states something along the lines of, "not to be used by those with liver disease"), but even in the first dose the drug is overwhelming the liver and restricting the liver from doing the job it was intended to do: removing foreign and toxic substances. As the liver gets backed up and can't remove enough junk, the body will often store this junk in fat cells, or deposit it into joints and tissues.

Think of it like that episode of *I Love Lucy* when Lucy is working in the chocolate factory on the conveyor belt. As the chocolate starts to come in faster than she has the ability to keep up, she starts to cram the chocolate in her mouth, pockets, hat, anywhere she can find a safe place. If the body left junk in your bloodstream, it could disrupt the delicate balance and you could literally die. Since the balance of the bloodstream is so important, the body wouldn't let that extreme imbalance happen so it just stores bad stuff in fat cells or other tissues and plans on coming back later to remove it when the coast is clear. Unfortunately, with our taking meds consistently and constantly punching our liver in the mouth, along with all the junk we put in our bodies, the coast is never clear and we can begin to swell like the Stay Puft Marshmallow Man as we accumulate stored water, fat or toxicity in places where it should not be. So, when we gain weight, it is actually our body's way of saving our life. Now, weight gain does have its own health dangers when it becomes excessive, but isn't it smarter for the body to gain weight until the excess weight causes a problem over the choice of dying this Thursday because of all the toxins left in the bloodstream? This is only one possible cause for weight gain. Read my upcoming book, *Kick Your Fat in the Nuts* to learn more. You can also watch clips from my documentary, *Why Am I So Fat?*, by visiting the website at: www.WhyAmISoFatMovie.com. This film will be released in 2013.

As far as why we are told to take these meds and why it often seems like the best option, that's something you can decipher for yourself with a new understanding of how money moves through the marketplace. People tend to do what they're paid to do. Our effort here is to help you do what will benefit you. We're not trying to explain to you why pharmaceutical products are not in your best interest. That's really not our agenda. Our intention is to do the right thing, not to try to justify why we're doing the right thing or to bash the guys who might be doing the wrong thing. If a person has enough time to make good decisions, he can make decisions that help him qualify to not need drugs. Some people don't have that much time; some people need drugs. Some don't. We're here to help the ones who have enough time to have options and are willing to do the work to make those options effective. Some people are not willing to do the work and that's okay. If you fit into the category of people who are not willing to do the work, you might find that this book can still function very well as a coaster to set your beer on while you watch *America's Next Top Model.*

In moving forward, I want to make sure you understand how the medical world operates so you don't have to be confused or frustrated when you see conflicting information. The best route to go, in my opinion, is to investigate the things that seem intriguing or appear as if they might turn out to make some sense. Just put your health back in your hands so you can work with your doctor, or health care practitioner, on issues that arise instead of counting on them to figure out the causes behind your health issues in the 16 minutes that they spend with you during your office visit. I mean really. Last week, I got more attention from "Habeeb" selling me a camera at Best Buy than I ever have from my doctor. There are a lot of people who absolutely love to slam the medical community for operating this way, but I think it's important to take a step back, get realistic, and be honest about why the medical "market" works the way it does.

To share these thoughts I wrote a chapter that includes more thoughts and funny stories on how the medical world operates (some were a little too funny for this book) and you can read it at:

www.KickItInTheNuts.com. I felt this info should be shared with everyone for free so I added this chapter to my site instead of putting it in my books. Just click on "Hidden Chapter." We've even set it up so you can email this "Hidden Chapter" to a friend for free.

Do I Qualify To Read This Book?

I feel that if you bought this book, you qualify to read it. Not in the sense that, "I paid for this, so I can read it." I just mean that if you're someone who is proactive enough in your search for knowledge that you're taking the time to dig for answers, you're the type of person I want reading my books. For you to take the time and effort involved in initiating your own quest, it's likely you have tried medical avenues in the past that failed and the lack of solutions available is beginning to bore you. I applaud you for your willingness to be a contestant in your own game of health, instead of merely hoping someone can figure out your woes for you. Not everyone, however, is as open as you are to this type of journey.

A lot of people who are sick, or struggling with their health, have been paying into the world of hospitalization and medical insurance for the last twenty years at the rate of $500-$800 per month. When you try to explain to some of these people that they need to pay money out-of-pocket to see a professional who is not covered by insurance, or buy supplements that don't fall under their medical plan, many will say, "Hey, I get all this stuff for free from my medical doctor." For these folks, it can be very hard to pay out-of-pocket because that validates that they may have been incorrectly spending $500-$800 per month for most of their life. It's almost as if people are invested in the American Medical Association (AMA) and they just want to see things work out since they have dumped so much money into that system. It reminds me of that miserable relationship where you really want it to work out because the sex is great and you really like his Mom. But how long do you stay with a tool-bag who's never had

20

a job and only showers on Thursdays, before you realize that he's a waste of flesh?

Even if you are a person who has been beaten up and left for dead by the medical world, and you have an understanding that you can't just use drugs to cover up a symptom and truly improve your health, recognizing why some people are resistant to anything that falls outside of the AMA will make your life much easier. When I first began learning how the body really works, I wanted to save the world and tell everyone I knew how they could fix the problems that have been plaguing them. Let me save you some trouble by telling you that's not your job. The best thing you can do for a loved one is to improve your own health and lead by example. I get a lot of people who tell me, "You need to see my uncle. His health is horrible." Well, I don't want to see your uncle unless he seeks me out. If you drag your loved ones into a party they didn't want to go to in the first place, they're going to have a lousy time and puke all over the coffee table. Think of it this way, if a baby wakes from a nap on his own accord, he will cry a little bit and then he will be a happy baby. But if *you* try to wake a baby while he's still in a deep sleep, you're going to have a calamity on your hands. You will learn very quickly not to do that again.

While you read this book and become excited about the possibilities for your sister, or your husband, or your neighbor who can't stop peeing himself, realize that it is not your job to save the world. You do qualify to read this book because you are awake to the possibilities. You are awake to the fact that you are responsible for your own health. Not everyone is that conscious. Remember that so you can avoid waking any sleeping babies. As a fellow human with a new piece of knowledge, your job is to simply sort through the people you know who could benefit from this information and separate those who still believe in Santa Claus from those who don't. I explain this here because you will find a lot of scoop in this book that, frankly speaking, is going to be very refreshing to you. To have these realities explained in a way that makes sense will be a new experience for many, when it comes to health topics. In that regard, when you try to share this information with your friends, it will be helpful to understand why they may be resistant. That doesn't mean that you can't help yourself tremendously with this insight. It just means that your friend has not been beaten up enough to be in a position to search for real answers yet. That's okay. You are and that's why you're here.

How To Use This Knowledge

When looking at the body from a natural point of view, as my colleagues and I do, two of the primary factors we focus on are urine and saliva. Urine is the trash can of life, that's what you're throwing out. Saliva is what you're holding on to. Saliva can give you a clue of what the fluid is like between the cells (otherwise known as the intercellular fluid). When you compare what is being thrown out by the urine against what's being held onto by the saliva, you can start to get some discernment about what's going on, and that's how we begin to get a picture of how the body is operating. This can be very enlightening because urine and saliva are not compensated fluids like the blood (I will explain this further a little later). The body doesn't hold on to the urine saying, "Oh, I can't pee this, what if someone sees it?" No, it absolutely goes out and we can collect information from what is going out. That's why it's a viable method to understand how a body is operating. By viewing this comparison, along with other physiological measurements like breath rate, blood pressure, and pulse (explained in chapter four), you will begin to see how natural health professionals can use this information to build a picture of what's needed for the wellness of an individual.

That's not to say that if you have Addison's Disease, or some of these really grievous diseases, that you don't need a doctor. That's not to say that if you cut off a finger you're not going to go down to the hospital and get it sewn back on. These are things that need to be handled by professionals. But just like you can check the oil

22

in your car, and you can check the water level, and you're expected to do these cursory things to try to avoid breaking down on the side of the road, so it is with what I'm teaching you to do in this book. You will learn to check a few things and avoid some health problems. When my colleagues and I work as natural health professionals, we're not trying to replace medicine. We think people should go to the doctor, and have a relationship with the doctor, and we don't think we're the alternative. We think we're the complement. We simply want to educate people so they can walk into their doctor's office and have an intelligent conversation and participate in their own health. We're the adjudicative, we're the additional, we're the helper to people who are conscious. We're not trying to replace anything. Ultimately, we are all going to need a doctor. What we'd like to do is need one in the last week of life, not the last seven years of life. So that's what you're doing with this book. You're lifting the hood saying, "Let's take a look at this, see what's going on and see what can be done."

Now, if you drive a Volkswagen Bug and that car gets totaled by a Bug Exterminator truck (yes, that happened to me in high school), you're not going to "look under the hood" and fix that much damage. You need to have the same viewpoint here. If you're dealing with breast cancer right now, don't think that you're going to "look under the hood" and make that go away. You're going to need professional help. But if your "car" is running a little funny or making some noise, the knowledge you can find in this book may be enough to help you get it running more smoothly.

You have an opportunity here to begin understanding how your specific body is operating. You may even be able to recognize some imbalances that you are experiencing and you may even find some food, nutrition or lifestyle changes that could help improve those imbalances. Just be sure to understand that the body is very complicated and, in most cases, if a person is really trying to improve a severe symptom, condition, or even something more serious, that individual is going to need some help from a professional who has a firm grasp on these foundational principles. So, don't try to be a hero and figure it all out yourself. There really is no reason to show off in that way and you will much more likely just create added frustration for yourself. We're going to teach you what to look at and even where you can find tools to chart your progress and monitor your changes on your own, but we're also going to show you where you can find help when you need it, so be sure you understand how much time and effort you will save by finding a professional to help you along.

Even though you may have a particular symptom that you are looking to relieve, when people first start to learn how their bodies are functioning, it is important to understand that we are all in submission to the intelligence of the body. While people may want relief from their "poor vision" or "skin irritation," we cannot dictate to the body what is to be its priority in the sequence of healing. If the kidneys are shutting down and about to fail, but you really wish you had a six-pack, the body is going to put its attention on helping the dying kidneys. While the "cries for relief" (or cries for a tighter butt) do not fall upon deaf ears, understanding the agricultural reality of the earth that we are part of is important. As people begin to balance their bodies, the body will dictate which areas will see the improvement first. This mentality separates us from practicing "plastic surgery medicine" that is only looking to change the exterior without any effect on the interior.

It's important to understand that people need to take responsibility for their own health. Most people will not be able to simply take a few supplements, or remove a few foods from their diet, and correct every issue that may have been developing for the last two or three decades. You will, however, be able to watch your chemistry and see if you are moving in the right direction, even before you might notice any changes in how you feel. For many, improved chemistry is often enough to keep them on track long enough to reap the rewards. In the "throwing darts" approach that is often used, in the natural world as much as the medical world, people will often begin using the right approach that will correct the imbalance that is causing their underlying problem. But since this approach doesn't bring about an immediate "drug-like" response, they stop or move on to the next big thing. When looking to help your body correct its own issues, keep in mind that this process will take much longer than the 4-6 hours it often takes for a drug to kick in. In nature, things that happen fast are often bad things. The best things happen slowly. A flower doesn't wake up and go, "BAM!!!" open. The flower opens very slowly and gradually. The sun doesn't just appear out of nowhere in full force. That would freak us out every single time. The sun rises gradually, just as it sets, just as the grass grows and the seasons change. Let your body do the same. If you're looking to "fix" a problem by Friday because you don't want it to interfere with the big square dance you hope to attend, you're going to find yourself very frustrated. Not only because you really need a better social life if a square dance is your big event, but also because you're setting yourself up for failure if you believe you can change the agriculture of your body in a few days. You can't.

Testing Tools You'll Need For This Book

In chapter four, we're really going to dig in to self-testing and how to look at your own chemistry and get a picture of how your body is operating. I just want to touch on some tools that will be helpful so you can get a hold of them before you get to that section of the book. These tools can normally be found and ordered on the website, www.NaturalReference.com, but can also be found at just about any drug store and/or health food store in your area.

• pH Testing Strips
Some drug stores will carry these and most health food stores will keep them in stock. Just don't let them sell you other "alkalizing" products when they see you picking up pH testing strips. There is

a LOT of bad information out there about pHs, so don't waste your time on that frontier like I did. You'll learn the truth about pHs in this book. A package or roll of pH strips will usually run between $10-18. Health store clerks also sell a lot of ketone strips to those on the Atkins Diet so be sure they don't send you home with ketone strips when you ask for pH strips.

• Glucometer

This is a great tool to own and every household in the country should have one. The glucometer will always be sold separately from the strips because the strips expire, whereas the glucometer does not. You can find a glucometer pretty cheap these days, but the strips can cost around $50 for a pack of 50. If you have friends who are diabetic, ask them if you can use their glucometer one morning before you eat anything. If you find that your blood sugar is in a good range, you might be able to go without this tool for a while if you need to budget things out.

• Blood Pressure Cuff

This is a pretty important tool if you're experiencing cramps, and one I would recommend buying. The money you spend will be well worth having the ability to monitor your progress. You can get a good one for around $50. You won't know if you're on the right track without one. I like the push-button style that does all the work for you and has a strap that is easy to put on yourself. You can look at the styles on www.NaturalReference.com to see examples of acceptable units. It usually does not matter which one you get, as long as you have a way to see if you're improving or if you need to make adjustments. The wrist types are okay too, but generally not as accurate and seem to run a little low on the reading. You could take it with you to your doctor's office and when they check your blood pressure, you can check your machine as well so you can compare and know how much to adjust your reading at home. Many drug stores will also have those big sit-down machines that allow you to check your blood pressure. These are suitable if a blood pressure cuff is not in your budget, but it sure is nice to be able to check your blood pressure at home when you need to.

- Stop Watch

You can also use a common digital kitchen timer or anything with a second hand. Or, I am also pretty sure there is an app for that.

There are other tools I may suggest as we go along, but the tools above are the main things you will need to "get to know yourself."

CHAPTER TWO

What's With The Cramps?

If this issue has been bugging you for a while now, you've likely searched the Internet for answers. Chances are, you've heard about hormones, prostaglandins, and "It's just your uterus contracting." Once you understand the variety of problems that can cause cramps, I have a feeling you're going to be a little upset that nobody has supplied you with the information I'm about to share. Take your time and let these ideas soak in. Don't just rush through looking for the quick answer that may apply to you. It's too easy to miss something and end up having to come back and read through it again.

The point I drive home throughout this book is this: With just about any symptom, there can be multiple causes. Some symptoms can be more serious than others. Some may be easier to improve. Some may not apply to you at all. It's likely that I'll cover topics that will have you thinking, "What the heck does this have to do with my cramps? Why can't this idiot just get to the point?" Remember that this book is about improving health and not about fighting or beating one problem. The body is a complex machine, even more complex than an Etch-a-Sketch. (I'm really good at making the stairs.) Many issues and imbalances can have layers of causes that all need to be addressed. In that same manner, one little imbalance can throw five or six systems out of whack, and if you can improve that one imbalance, all kinds of craziness can go back to normal.

I feel that it is important for you to understand the causes behind the causes. Understanding will make it easier and more motivating to do the work to improve those underlying causes. Answers to your "whys" can also reduce anxiety and remove that "why does this happen to me" feeling. In this chapter, we're going to talk about what causes cramps, why some people get them and other lucky little bitches don't, how mineral and nutrient assimilation can be involved, and how long it might take for you to begin seeing some relief. The sooner you understand that you can't just hold the Etch-a-Sketch upside down and shake it to get rid of your cramps, the easier this journey will be. I hope you're ready, because it's about to get jazzy.

What Causes Cramps?

Make an effort to move your thinking beyond the normal "what is causing this" mindset. Below, I'm going to dig into some of the underlying causes that can bring about those nasty cramps. As you read them, however, be mindful that just because an issue *can* create cramps doesn't mean that is the cause behind *your* cramps. Cramps often result from a combination of circumstances and that combination can be different for each person. I'm going to talk about digestion and how this one factor is the most common underlying cause for menstrual cramps. Nonetheless, the reasons that a person may be having digestive issues, or how those issues are manifesting trouble in the body, can be different for everyone. With that in mind, stick around and work your way through this whole book before you start jumping to conclusions. I'm going to show you how to look at *you,* instead of picking which cause you *believe* is the root of your trouble.

Everything Goes Back To Digestion

Odds are pretty great that you will be surprised to learn, in nearly every case of menstrual cramps, it all goes back to digestion. Now, don't look at this like I'm saying you ate something that didn't sit well in your stomach and gave you cramps. (Although, that would be hilarious if some guy wrote a whole book on cramps because he thought girls were just experiencing more indigestion and that's what girls meant when they talked about cramps. Hopefully, I'm not that dumb.) When I talk about digestion, I'm talking about people's ability to properly break down the foods they are eating. In life, we tend to think that if food goes in one end and poop comes out the other, everything is working as planned. That is not always the case. Digestive issues are actually much more common than one might think. To illustrate: Line up 100 high school boys. You will likely find that the percentage of guys whose pants do not fit properly coincides with the percentage of people in this country who have some type of digestive issue. I know! That's a really high percentage. (And why don't they buy pants that fit... why?)

Diet is what a person eats but nutrition is what the cells see. Let me repeat that sentence. (Actually, I'm trying to save some space here so would you mind just going back and reading that sentence again? It's that important and I'd rather use this space for other information. Thank you.) Nutrition not making it to the cells is where we find the big disconnect. People think that if they focus on foods that are higher in specific nutrients, calcium for example, they're improving their calcium levels with these food choices. Little do they realize, if the body can't properly break down the food they are eating into nutrients that can be used by the body, they're just treating their toilets to calcium-rich poop. Meanwhile, these people truly are trying to do right by themselves and putting in the effort for the good fight, yet they are still left wondering why their efforts aren't paying off.

In order for digestion to function properly, there are processes that MUST be in place or all the nutrients can't be pulled out of the food we eat. In chapter seven I talk in more detail about digestion and how it works. Just know that this is huge. Correcting these digestive issues, if they exist for you, can improve a whole lot more than cramps.

Why Am I Getting Cramps? My Friend Never Gets Cramps.

Women don't get cramps because "all the cool kids get them." "If your friends jumped off a cliff, would you jump too?" (If I had a nickel for every time my mom asked me that, every store I went into, the employees would say, "Great, here comes the guy that pays with all nickels.") Cramps are not socially selective. They don't gravitate to one group of friends and leave another group of friends alone. Each woman is her own person. Each individual has unique chemistry that is likely different from nearly every other person in the world—much like a fingerprint. It's even comparable to the way no two *Shrinky Dinks* will turn out exactly the same once you bake them. That's what's missing from health care in the world today: Instead of looking at the individual, the typical medical professional is just treating symptoms according to what you bitch about the loudest. But if we look at the chemistry of an individual, we can begin to get an idea of what issues may be causing those cramps in that individual. That would explain how one girl can have no cramps while the other girl is balled up in the fetal position on the floor of the ladies' restroom at Target.

One girl has a body chemistry that is predisposed to create an environment where cramps are abundant, while the other girl's body is operating in a manner that prevents that from happening. In my opinion, this is not a curse that you are just stuck with. You can get stuck with a brother that constantly hits on all your friends even though he has no shot—there's not much you can do about that. You were really just born into that situation. It is much easier to control body chemistry than it is a schmuck brother. When it comes to cramps, many women are able to move their chemistry and adjust some systems to improve the discomfort—or eliminate it all together.

All Cramps Are Not Created Equal

Though the basic process that the body goes through during a menstrual cycle is the same design for every woman, the discomfort that can be experienced from woman to woman can vary drastically. How is that fair? Why would that be the case if the process is basically the same for all girls who have a menstrual cycle? The difference is almost always the resources that each body has at its disposal to complete this process.

Imagine this: You and your friend are each building a birdhouse. In front of you we find a do-it-yourself birdhouse kit, complete with all the pre-cut wood pieces, nails, screws, a hammer and screwdriver—everything you need to put it together. They even threw in a little bag of birdseed. It's basically like an IKEA birdhouse, so you'll end up with a few extra screws and pieces that you have no idea where the hell they go, but it will still be very easy to put together.

Your friend, on the other hand, has a pile of wood and some duct tape. As the two of you build your birdhouses, it doesn't take long before your dwelling begins to take shape. There are even spring robins eyeing it from a tree nearby. The horrifying variety of obscenities flailing from your friend's mouth suddenly brings your attention to her project where she is currently trying to wipe off the blood gushing from her hand. She was doing okay until she tried to wedge two pieces of wood together since she doesn't have any nails.

Upon completion, yours looks like a birdhouse. IKEA would be proud. Your friend's birdhouse, on the other hand, looks like the *Deathstar*, mid-explosion. The strands of duct tape hanging from each perch end up working like giant, industrial fly-paper, creating a massacre of a deathtrap for any bird that visits. Children cry as they watch little birdies trying to flap away from the grip of the duct tape and this becomes the main topic of the next Homeowner's Association meeting. The moral of the story is: If you don't have the right resources to complete a project correctly, not only is the process going to be very painful and discomforting, but the whole mess can end up causing other problems as well.

In addition to discussing why one individual may be lacking the resources to get through a menstrual cycle with little to no discomfort, I will also touch on how trying to complete this cycle without enough resources can cause problems in other areas for the body too. Poor, poor little birdies.

To understand menstrual cramps, let's first take a good look at (1) muscle cramps (2) how muscles and tissues work, and (3) how different minerals can play a role in how muscles and tissues function.

Muscle Cramps And Calcium

Have you ever had a charley horse? Son of a sack-a-nuts, that hurts. I'm talking about those cramps you get in your calf or feet, especially while you're sleeping. What the french, Toast? It feels like somebody stuck a car battery to your leg while you were asleep, just to see how high you would fly off the bed. You jump up and immediately start punching your leg to try to make the cramp go away. Those are less than fun, so let's try to understand why this happens.

Calcium in the tissues is the mineral that allows your muscles to relax once they have contracted. Magnesium can be involved too, but the main mineral in this process is calcium. If your tissues do not contain the proper amount of calcium, once your muscles contract, they can get stuck since there is not enough calcium to let

33

that muscle relax, annnnnd... cramp. When it comes to menstrual cramps, issues with magnesium and even iron can exist. But since it is most commonly a problem of low calcium at the tissue level, I'm going to focus on that for a bit while I'm talking about muscle cramps. Now, don't run out and buy some calcium and think that you're going to fix the problem. You may already have plenty of calcium in the system and, for one reason or another (most of which I will cover in this book), that calcium is not in the right place.

I can't say that the calcium in our tissues is the most important calcium we have. After all, bones are pretty important; without them, we would be just a blob on the floor. If humans were built this way, I fear that whole break-dancing phase in the eighties could have been lost altogether, and who wants a world where *Breakin' 2: Electric Boogaloo* never existed? Outside of our bones, however, I do feel that the calcium in the tissues is the most important calcium we have. As soon as calcium deficiencies start to show up at the tissue level, it can be just like an episode of *Three's Company*, where new trouble seems to show up every day.

Calcium And The Overrated Vitamin D

I'm going to get up on a soapbox for a minute, but it's only because I'm not very tall. Vitamin D may be one of the biggest mistakes ever made by the medical world. Vitamin D is the nutrient that allows us to move calcium from the intestines into the bloodstream, so we are very grateful for that. Otherwise, we would not be able to pull calcium from our food into the system. Be that as it may, the medical world tells us that we need huge doses of vitamin D to assimilate calcium because that's what their clinical trials came up with. In a clinical trial, they test people's calcium levels in the blood (instead of digging into their bones because who would sign up for that?) Then they give those people vitamin D and test their blood for calcium again. Since the calcium level goes up after use of vitamin D, that means the vitamin D helps them assimilate more calcium, right? Nope. It's actually almost the opposite. When talking about vitamin D, it's important to separate correlation from causation. This can be likened to our view of a fever. It appeared a fever always developed when someone was sick, so we used to correlate a fever to sickness. We now know that to be wrong. The fever is the immune response to the sickness and is part of the cure. There is a correlation between sickness and fever, but the fever is not the cause of the sickness as used to be thought in early days, before we had parachute pants.

I mentioned how vitamin D helps calcium make the jump from the intestinal tract into the bloodstream, but if you walk outside in the sun for a few minutes your body makes its own vitamin D. In higher doses (like we're now being told to take), it not only pulls the calcium out of the intestines into the bloodstream, like it is intended to do, it also starts to pull calcium out of the tissues AND BONES and then holds the calcium in the bloodstream. Vitamin D makes the blood calcium-retentive, meaning that now the calcium can't leave the bloodstream and go down to the tissue level where it can be utilized.

Think of vitamin D as a Dust Buster that sucks calcium out of the intestinal tract. If you increase your levels of vitamin D as high as mainstream medicine is suggesting, that Dust Buster would turn into an industrial sized Shop-Vac, sucking up calcium from every direction.

Yes, vitamin D has some beneficial uses in the body, but when we get it in high amounts, it could cause much more trouble than good. In high doses, vitamin D pulls calcium out of where it's supposed to be and holds it in the bloodstream. I've already talked about how calcium leaving the tissues can create cramps, but let's cover what other kinds of fun prizes we can see when the calcium that belongs in the tissues begins to leave those tissues and can be held hostage in the bloodstream.

Dr. Royal Lee founded Standard Process, one of the largest distributors of quality supplements sold only through health care practitioners. He was one of the early pioneers to understand that a lack of calcium at the tissue level can affect our immune system. Mark Anderson (a natural health expert who travels the world educating doctors and health care professionals about nutrition) has a great recorded lecture called, *The Triad: Dr. Royal Lee and the Immune System.* It's an excellent explanation of the many purposes of calcium at the tissue level. The most important factor to understand when it comes to calcium and the immune system is this: Calcium in our tissues is what triggers our immune system to attack. Without that calcium in the tissues, it's almost as if the immune system doesn't even know invaders exist. This is sort of like that guy who wears a Speedo at the beach and doesn't even understand how much he looks like a tool. In the same way the normal "be a reasonable human" signal doesn't get to his Speedo-wearing brain, without calcium at the tissue level, the warning that there are intruders doesn't seem to make it to our immune system.

I have a perfect example. If you get a fancy herpes-style cold sore, we know it was created by a virus. But as long as you have enough calcium at the tissue level, that virus can't flower and you don't get any cold sores. I've seen this a hundred times. A client will be getting cold sores regularly, and once the steps are taken to make calcium available at the tissue level, those cold sores just stop. You might see similar results with someone who seems to catch every virus that walks by. Once the calcium is in the tissues, so the immune system can be notified to attack intruders, those viruses don't take over anymore. It really is incredible to see. On the downside, pushing calcium back down to the tissue level doesn't seem to knock any sense into the brain of the Speedo-wearing circus freak.

There is some good news about vitamin D for a person who has low mineral content. When this person takes vitamin D, the calcium that gets pulled out of the tissues can thicken up the blood, raise the blood pressure, and that individual who had low mineral content and low blood pressure will often feel and function better. That's why a lot of girls with low blood pressure love to tan. They feel great afterwards. If you were to do this, however, you'd be mining your body of what it needs, and where it needs to be, in order to get this "feel better" result. Yes, you're taking a mineral and thickening up the blood, but you're doing so basically by stealing that mineral from your tissues and even from your bones.

That's why, even though mainstream medicine tells us how important vitamin D is to fight osteoporosis, osteoporosis has been on the rise ever since they've been telling us that. Vitamin D is actually the perfect recipe for osteoporosis. We know we need calcium to build bones. Since mainstream thinking says that vitamin D helps us assimilate more calcium, why wouldn't that help fight osteoporosis? It's understandable why they would think that when you look at their view of how vitamin D works. However, with your new understanding of what is really going on with vitamin D, it's easy to understand how high doses of vitamin D are truly the perfect formula to pull calcium out of the bones, into the bloodstream and make those bones weaker.

Once excess vitamin D pulls calcium out of the tissues and holds it in the bloodstream, the bloodstream will have all this calcium floating around which means: If the kidneys are unable to excrete the higher calcium precipitated by the excess vitamin D, the body, overwhelmed by too much calcium in the bloodstream, will allow some of the calcium to be deposited in the joints. Do you know anybody with joint pain? I'm not saying this is the only cause of joint pain, it's not. But the pain that comes along with calcification of the joints can be about as fun as eating Cheerios with a slingshot. (Wait, that does sound sort of fun. Painful, but fun.)

Did you know vitamin D is actually utilized as a rat poison? Of the calcium that floats around the system, some is bound to protein and some is not bound to protein. It's the calcium that is not bound to protein that causes the trouble. Since rats have low protein, the higher levels of vitamin D will raise their blood calcium (the kind not bound to protein) to dangerous levels that will cause kidney failure. Dead rat. I don't want to imply that the dosage of vitamin D used to kill a rat is comparable to what is given to people; body weights differ significantly unless you're talking about a very small person or a big honkin' rat.

Even with that understanding, we are still told that the reason vitamin D is bad for rats is the same reason that it's good for us... because we have more protein. But what about people whose digestion is not properly breaking down proteins and their protein levels are very low? Wouldn't that make excessive vitamin D levels just like rat poison for those people? This is not at all a "clinical fact," but most of the women I see with real cramp issues are having these problems because their digestion is not working well enough to bring in sufficient mineral. If digestion is not working well enough to bring in needed mineral, it's usually not breaking down protein very well either. With this line of thinking, if you are reading this book because you have cramps, I would sooner punch you in the face before I told you to take high doses of vitamin D.

To watch a great, two-minute video that illustrates how vitamin D works, go to www.KickItInTheNuts.com and click on BOOK VIDEOS.

Why Did Blood Tests Tell Me I Had Low Vitamin D?

When a person's blood tests come back saying that vitamin D is low, the medical world just looks at the average numbers and says, "Oh, I see his level is lower, he must need more D." Why not stop to think WHY the body may be restricting vitamin D production? Doesn't it make sense that, if a person already had a high level of calcium in the bloodstream and lower levels of calcium at the tissue level, then the body may appropriately reduce the amount of vitamin D being produced because it doesn't want to pull MORE calcium out of the tissues and into the bloodstream? Why would the body want to take more calcium out of the tissues, where it belongs, and put it into the blood where levels may already be too high?

We've already discussed how the calcium in our tissues is pretty much the most important calcium we have. To keep the body from stripping tissues of needed calcium, the body will produce less vitamin D. People are told to cram more in but you can see that the body's intentions are good. The body understands that the opposite is required to bring about balance. Do you remember Beaker from The Muppets? Do you remember how he looked like an idiot no matter what he did? This is what I picture when I think of the scientific world running an experiment in a petri dish and believing the outcome will be the same in the human body. It won't. Don't be a Beaker.

It is not until a person's vitality diminishes to the point that she is no longer controlling electrical, chemical and biological processes that the petri dish mentality can be applied to the human. When the body has given up control, what happens on the lab bench will also happen in the body. But until then the body's own control mechanisms are the very identity of the entity—bringing about individuality.

Vitamin D And Heart Health

The conclusion that vitamin D is good for heart health comes from a similar "let's be sure we don't think with our brain" approach. The studies basically show that people with low vitamin D are more likely to have heart disease, or a heart attack or stroke. The conclusion derived from this piece of information is, "Just give them more vitamin D since the people with low vitamin D keep having heart attacks." That's like saying, people make stupid decisions while they're drunk. Therefore, if you eliminate alcohol, you will remove all stupidity from the planet. Since the creators of the motion picture, *Battlefield Earth*, were not drunk during production, we know this to be inaccurate. The medical world is not looking at circumstances; they're just looking at clinical trial statistics. I will talk about these clinical trials in a moment, but let's dig deeper into this heart health issue first. (I won't dig deeper into the stupidity issue here because that's a whole other book.)

You'll soon be able to read more about high blood pressure in *Kick High Blood Pressure in the Nuts*, but to present a very vague overview of a high blood pressure issue, I will say this: High blood pressure is commonly a situation where, for one reason or another, an individual is having trouble removing excess minerals or junk from the body. As a result, this "junk" begins to thicken the blood and raise an individual's blood pressure to a level that is seen as "too high." There are obviously many more details that go into looking at each individual and the different causes of high blood pressure, but this very vague explanation is enough to help us understand why vitamin D is not always such a great idea for people with heart complications.

If we understand that high blood pressure is commonly a thickening of the blood, we can see that giving vitamin D to a person with high blood pressure may not be ideal. In spite of the fact that vitamin D acts as a vascular relaxant, the calcium being pulled into the bloodstream is just further thickening the blood, causing the kidneys to be more and more overwhelmed and creating even greater risk for heart problems.

A fact frequently overlooked in the medical world is that calcium follows sugar (high blood sugar seems to act like vitamin D making the bloodstream calcium retentive), and all of these people who have high heart risks commonly have high sugar and high insulin levels. So, their bodies would already be pulling calcium out of the tissues and holding it in the bloodstream because of all the high sugars. Of course the body would make less vitamin D in this situation, since pulling more calcium into the bloodstream would just make the problem worse.

Most blockages consist of cholesterol and calcium. That combination is what the body uses as a type of "Spackle" to repair damages from high insulin levels. By taking vitamin D for "heart health," we're really giving our bodies more tools to clog things up. Seriously, our great grandkids are just going to point and laugh. I know it seems unbelievable that we would make such incredible mistakes, but keep in mind that people in this country used to think it was a good idea to drown someone suspected of being a witch. If the woman didn't drown, she was a witch and would be executed. If she did drown, she wasn't a witch and everything was okay. Oh yeah, except that she was dead. Well, at least everyone knew she wasn't a witch.

Clinical Trials

A new clinical trial reported recently that high blood pressure rates would drop 68% if they would put *Alf* back on the air. I'm pretty sure I'm the only person who has ever written that statement, but it makes my point that we will believe just about anything that was discovered by a clinical trial. It's my opinion that these clinical trials are often the origin of bad information. Once you understand how every individual is different, and no two people have the same chemistry, or are able to process foods, emotions or pollutants the exact same way, we begin to see that giving a room full of people the same supplement, drug, or forcing them all to wear a Fonzie jacket, really doesn't prove anything.

When we look at results from a clinical trial, the only consistency we know across the board is that all participants were human. These days, it can even be hard to tell gender. (I learned that the hard way in Key West but I'd rather not talk about it.) We really don't know any of the important factors about these clinical trial participants. We don't know if they are digesting their food correctly. We don't know if they even have the ability to assimilate whatever substance they are testing. It's all a crapshoot. When the numbers turn out that 59% of headache sufferers improved when they ate a peanut butter and jelly sandwich at 5:30 P.M. every day, suddenly the world comes to a halt at 5:30 to spread a little Jif on some bread. What about the other 41% of the participants? Even if they experienced an increase in symptom severity, the trial still says PBJs help the majority of headache sufferers. Unless we're looking at a person's individual chemistry, and then taking stock of how a substance can move that chemistry while it creates changes to those symptoms, we're just cramming a hundred people in a dark closet, throwing in a Freddy Krueger mask, and then counting the number of people who pee their pants. How is this science?

The only thing we do know about a clinical trial is that it was bought and paid for by somebody. Some company (most often a pharmaceutical manufacturer) put up the money to fund this trial (and trials are not cheap) because they were hoping to create a specific result that would help them sell a drug, procedure or substance.

The lesson here about clinical trials is this: Even a Fonzie jacket can't make everybody look cool, and don't make decisions about your health based on the results of a group of people whose chemistry was unknown before the trial and remains unknown after the trial. Without a clear, chemistry-driven baseline to start from, how can you come to any conclusions about whatever it was they were testing?

I especially love the morality involved in the clinical trials that test new drugs. To take a group of sick people who are all hoping to improve their situation by using "this great new wonder-drug," and give the drug to only half of the people. Everyone else gets a placebo. How mean is that? Unless, of course, those running the trial understand that the chances are just as good that the drug will bring about more harm than benefit. How much do they pay people do to this? Union workers get "hazard pay," maybe that should be included in these trials as well. Analyses of these studies have actually shown that, more often than not, a placebo has a better "healing" track-record than any drug.

Calcium Following Sugar

Sugar intake alone is rarely the main cause for escalated cramps but can often be a contributing factor. Since I just mentioned calcium likes to follow sugar, let's look at how that can affect your cramps. For those of you who look at chocolate and sugar like they're crack, and you would sooner give up a foot before you considered reducing your sugar and chocolate intake, don't let this information freak you out. Later in this book, when I talk about cravings, I'll explain why you feel like you need these foods, some things you can do to reduce your "need" for them, and a few tricks that will reduce the negative result I'm about to explain to you. Just put down the lighter and don't burn the book merely because I mentioned reducing chocolate or sugar. Right now I am going to explain how they can increase your cramps, and then later I'll talk about how to improve these hurdles. Nice book. No fire needed.

You have likely noticed that your cravings for sugar and chocolate can skyrocket around your period. I've even had one client tell me that when she went into the 7-11 just before her period to buy her favorite chocolate, and they were out, she took the turban off the cashier's head and popped him with it. Don't mess with a woman's chocolate around her period. What are you, new?

Unfortunately for the cramps, when you eat sugar, calcium will leave the tissues and follow that sugar. The result is similar to the way vitamin D pulls calcium out of the tissues, but in this case, the calcium is following the sugar. Can you blame the calcium? Are you saying that you've never run down the street chasing the ice cream truck? No matter what the cause, calcium leaving the tissues can still leave those tissues depleted of calcium, and we know what that means. More cramps.

43

As if that wasn't enough bad news about sugar, you will also recall my talking about how tissue calcium relates to viruses. With calcium leaving the tissues, it opens the door for any virus to come in and set up camp. Not enough calcium at the tissue level equates to a compromised immune system response. You and I have heard our whole lives that sugar isn't good for us, now you get to understand one of the main reasons why. Sugar shuts off the immune system by pulling calcium out of the tissues. Why do you think cold and flu season starts right after Halloween? People always assume the change to colder weather dictates cold and flu season, but many believe it has more to do with sugar consumption.

If you know how to trick or treat like a pro, your bag of candy will last you through November, just in time for fifteen pies to show up on Thanksgiving. By the time you work through those pies, cookies and candy start to become plentiful for Christmas, champagne and parties for New Year's Eve, and a big box of chocolates for Valentine's Day. How does your body have time to move calcium back to the tissue level with this onslaught of sugar? For many people, it doesn't, and flu season hits them hard. I used to get a cold every three weeks, almost without fail. This went on for years. Now that I understand how to keep calcium where it is intended to be, it's been more than five years since I've had a single cold. I don't say that to brag, it just sort of works out that bragging happens naturally as I say it.

In chapters six and nine, when I cover more details about cravings, you'll understand why you may love sugar so tremendously, and why it makes you feel much better around your period. But now it's important to understand what sugar is doing in regard to calcium. Later, I'm going to teach you some tricks that can help your body push calcium back down to the tissue level. Yes, I will be a hero. For now, just understanding the various reasons why calcium can leave the tissues, and how your cravings for sugar could be a contributor to your cramps, might be a huge piece to the puzzle.

Joint Pain And Bone Spurs

"Joint pain? Hey Schmuck! How is this about cramps? Get back to the reason I bought this book before I punch you in the neck." I promise this will all come together and make more sense than you ever thought it could. I just want to go a step further and talk about what happens to this calcium when too much leaves the tissues. Some of this science can get a little complicated, so I'm going to try to keep it basic. Not because I think you're dumb, it just hurts my brain to think about it. Remember, I'm just a boy and boys are a lot more stupid than girls are.

If you've ever mixed salt into water, you've seen the salt dissolve to the point where it just looks like water. If you add too much salt, however, you find that some of that salt will fall to the bottom of the glass. This is called "salting out." Once the water reaches a certain level of salt, it can no longer absorb anymore salt and the excess will fall to the bottom. Calcium in the blood acts in a similar way. Dr. Melvin Page taught us that calcium will stay ionized (it will continue floating in suspension) if it stays within the proper ratio to the mineral phosphorus. If we find ten parts calcium to four parts phosphorus, that calcium can stay ionized and continue to stay in the bloodstream. If we find twelve parts calcium to four parts phosphorus, that would result in two parts calcium "salting out" and falling out of solution. That salted-out calcium will form into a structure similar to salt and now the body will deposit it somewhere. It can be different for every person, but this excess calcium is often deposited in joints or on bones, like a bone spur.

When we see joint pain, we can sometimes be looking at calcium that salted out and accumulated in joints over a period of time. So calcium leaving the tissues can cause a lot more trouble than severe cramps. It can cause a lot more trouble than turning off your body's immune system and its ability to attack invaders. When we look at what happens to that calcium if too much leaves the tissues, and there is more in the bloodstream than the bloodstream can hold in solution, we see that we can now experience a whole new kind of agony in the form of arthritic pain or bone spurs. I'll explain this more and teach ways to improve these issues when I release *Kick Arthritis in the Nuts*, but just this quick explanation gives a fuller picture of how important it can be to keep enough calcium down at the tissue level.

Of course, we can't get our blood calcium levels tested all the time, but Dr. Carey Reams taught his students that if urine pH goes over 6.4, stop any vitamin D use. He felt like urine pH higher than 6.4 was a good indication that unbound calcium was at a high enough level that it could start to cause some problems. In chapter four, I'm going to lay out specific methods for you to easily get a picture of where your chemistry is and what steps might be most appropriate for you to see some improvement. Stand clear. You're about to become a participant in your own health. Who'd a thunk? (The fact that I appropriately place the word "thunk" in one of my books just totally made my day.)

CHAPTER THREE

Blood Work, Body Chemistry And Imbalances

Blood Work And Working Symptomatically In The Medical And Natural Health Fields

A phrase that seems to be cemented in Western culture is "cause and effect." People refer to this phrase as a cornerstone of scientific thinking. However, the reciprocal of this phrase, "effect and cause," seems to be practiced more by the health care industry. That is, the person who has a certain symptom is pigeonholed, believing his symptom can only have the popularly believed cause. Of course, this is a grave error in a field where grave errors have grave consequences.

It's possible for a symptom to have many different causes that can be layered, and different individuals with the same symptom could easily be experiencing that symptom due to totally different causes. Measuring the metabolic pathways of each person can pinpoint the causes of the symptoms. Viewing a symptom without measurement of the metabolic pathways and working with inverted "effect and cause" thinking makes as much sense as believing that changing the hand on a barometer will change the weather.

Everything we've learned on television for years and years, and I mean more then a few decades, going back to Dr. Kildare and Dr.

Ben Casey, is that everything goes off of symptoms. Well, there is a reason everything goes off of symptoms in this country and that's because all our health care is done with blood work. This is an exaggerated way of saying it, but if you can stand up and take a breath, your blood is probably going to be in range on the blood test.

All the science in medicine is designed around handling blood work and using that blood work as the main indication for what steps to take. Altered blood has been studied and "scientific" papers have been written. When a person's blood work is in range, and is not showing any altered readings, then there is no more science. If the blood is altered, then the doctors know what to do next—according to the "scientific" papers.

Let's say a guy goes to the doctor. The blood work says he's still in range. But the doctor looks at him and sees that his gills are green and his eyes are rolling back into his head. Because the doctor is a good person and wants to help this guy, the doctor asks, "Where does it hurt?" The guy will explain, "Well, it's like this, Doc..." From this point forward, the doctor will be working off symptoms, not off science from the blood work.

The blood tests are measuring a compensated fluid. Blood is compensated by the body. Let me explain what I mean when I say compensated.

The bloodstream is so vital for proper bodily function that the system will beg, borrow and steal from other areas of the body to make sure the blood itself is in proper order. If the blood doesn't have enough calcium in it, there are hormones and mechanisms that will move the blood calcium level to where it needs to be. Even if digestion is not successful enough to bring in adequate calcium, the body can just melt calcium down from the bones. Maybe there's not enough protein in the system, well, we can pull that out of lung tissue. What if there's too much sugar in the system? We can start pumping sugar into the kidneys, through

48

the bladder, and drop the sugar level of the bloodstream that way. The body is very adept at compensating the bloodstream. So when the blood work is in range and doesn't show an obvious problem, that is saying the body is still strong enough to compensate, or control the biological chemistry and processes. You have the ability to pay off your American Express card with your MasterCard. When blood goes totally out of range, that means now you've maxed out all of your credit cards, everybody knows you have a bad credit rating, and now your blood has drifted.

When talking about blood work, what's a measurement that commonly goes out of range with blood? Sugar. How long could a person live with elevated blood sugar levels? A long time. The human body is an awesome mechanism and it is strong. During the gold rush days in 1849 there were guys who had a little money, they had horses, and they took off for California on horseback. There were also guys who didn't have anything and they pushed wheelbarrows to get to California. Guess who got there first... The guys pushing the wheelbarrows got there first because humans ate foods that were higher octane than grass. The horse had to rest for several days, whereas the guys just kept on going; especially if they thought there was a horse in front of them. Little did they know, the horse was behind them because it would have keeled over if it hadn't stopped to rest. Humans are quite freaky like that. We really are a very strong mechanism even though it is not always apparent when you listen to a man with a head cold. Why do most big strong men become such little bitches when we get sick? However, the human body truly has the ability to go on and on when it needs to.

My point is: When a measurement, like glucose, finally drifts out of range with the blood, it's usually something a person can continue living with for quite some time. Keep in mind that this is really an oversimplification and it favors a bias that I'm presenting here. When a measurement in your blood drifts out of range, that is probably the least important item to look at in your situation.

49

The body is not stupid, it does not let things go out of range that are going to kill you quick. It's just overwhelmed and, as priorities in the system change, it has to start dropping tasks that are lower on the priority list.

Now, that's not the way it always is. These are grandiose viewpoints. Yet, that is what often happens. When there is no science left to direct a doctor on how to help this patient, the most frequent answer is for that doctor to look at the symptoms. The medical world is not the only place where this happens. Most natural practitioners work off of symptoms as well. They just use natural substances to improve those symptoms instead of drugs, but they are still pigeonholing a client into a "diagnosis" based on the symptoms. When working in this manner, a practitioner might as well be asking the clients to throw darts at a "diagnosis dart board." At least with this option, clients might leave the doctor's office with a stuffed animal.

My co-authors and I care about symptoms. Symptoms can sometimes give us insight into how the body is operating. However, symptoms are not the guiding criteria in the decision process. Treating yourself off of your symptoms can often cause more harm than good.

Communicating With Your Doctor And Working With A Natural Practitioner

The human body is a crazy machine. If we look at it realistically, we can admit that there isn't a person on the planet who really understands every single thing about how a body is operating. We just don't know. We might think we do, but every time we're absolutely certain that we know how something is working, we bust it open and all this other "stuff" comes out. So, while the technological advances we humans have made are incredible, let's just "simma down" and get a grip on the fact that we still have a lot to learn.

With that understanding in mind, yes, by reading this book and following the strategies I lay out, you will be able to understand a whole lot about how your specific body is operating; but that doesn't mean you'll be able to "fix" it all. There are just too many layers and options for how people's chemistries can change the way their bodies are operating. Also, specific imbalances can interact with each other and change how other systems in the body are functioning So, be prepared to have answers to questions about your body that you have probably been wondering about for most of your life; but, if you're unable to correct certain imbalances on your own, also be prepared to get help from professionals in your area who have spent their careers studying and learning how the body really works. The only difference here will be, when you get help from a professional, you will still be a knowledgeable participant in your efforts. It won't be like a doctor just giving you some pills to take and then you come back in a month so he can see if your lips turned purple or not. With the knowledge you gain here, you will understand what you're trying to do, and you'll be able to monitor what is working and what isn't. In this way, you can be an active participant in your health. It gets pretty fun.

With the large number of people who are reducing their need for medications by changing their diet and using natural supplements, more and more doctors are opening up to the possibilities. I'm sure you can imagine how frustrating it must be for many doctors when they see their patients becoming worse instead of improving from the treatments they are prescribing. So when diabetic patients, for example, come in and show a lower blood glucose reading that resulted from a change in their diet, especially if it's 100 points lower, not many doctors will say, "Stop whatever you're doing." The majority of doctors got into this business to help people—so they will be excited to see improvement. That being said, if you are dealing with a major health issue and you see improvements in your health, just don't get cocky and think you can read a book and handle this on your own. You really do need to communicate with your doctor on your progress and let the doctor help you reduce any medication when the time is right. Don't try to do this on your own. You may have other issues that are not covered here. Your doctor may be working on those issues as part of his or her grand scheme, so keep your doctor on the same page at all times. Just because most doctors don't understand the methods laid out in this book doesn't mean they won't understand what to do with your medication levels when your health begins to improve.

Body Chemistry And Imbalances

There are many sides to the natural health world. Some natural practitioners base their protocols on symptoms, just like the medical world. At the end of the day, these natural practitioners are just throwing darts or using Ouija boards like most doctors, or unskilled mechanics, often do (I once saw a commercial with a mechanic muscle testing a car for bad brakes). The only difference is that their darts are herbs, vitamins and other natural tools; so their darts are much less toxic, have fewer side effects and won't knock your liver into next week. Still, if a practitioner is treating symptoms and not the person, that practitioner is going to have, at best, a 50/50 chance of helping that individual correct most issues, since one person's symptom/condition can have a different underlying cause than a friend that has the same symptom/condition.

Another side of the natural health world looks at the chemistry of the person to get a better idea of what the cause may be for that individual. This is the side of natural health we are talking about in this book.

The medical world loves to come up with new names for "diseases" or "conditions." If they can name a problem that you're dealing with, you can be diagnosed. If you can be diagnosed, they can prescribe you a specific drug. We, as patients, generally feel better when there is a name for what has been ailing us and we find out we're not just a circus freak. "It's actually a real thing that other people deal with too," we say. Unfortunately, this is a fictional way of looking at health. Take Type II Diabetes for example. Type II Diabetes is not a disease that you can catch, or that you were even born with. It's just the name given by the medical world to a body when it is unable to properly process glucose. It is not, however, a "disease" that a person needs to fight and conquer, unless of course you're talking to an HMO where disease is a business. There are functional issues at play that have likely developed over years, or decades, that are now causing the body to operate in this manner. In most cases, a person can work on and improve these issues if the person is willing to put forth the effort. After all, Type II Diabetics across the globe are becoming "un-diabetic" every day by taking steps to correct these imbalances and the actual underlying causes that create this "disease."

You will be able to read more about how Type II Diabetics have improved their situations naturally when *Kick Type II Diabetes in the Nuts* hits the market. In the book you're reading now, I explain the ten major imbalances that most frequently occur in the body. These are the imbalances that seem to be responsible for just about any issue a person can experience. The degrees at which these imbalances show up are different for every person, and one imbalance can be layered on top of two or three others to create a very complicated picture of how that person's body is operating. I explain the basics here, but understand that most people who are dealing with significant issues will need the help of a professional to work through improving a lot of these imbalances. The variations that can occur are too numerous and intricate for this book to recount in detail. Having said that, the foundations you learn here will help you better communicate with a health care professional if your particular health issues are too complex for you to get a clear picture on your own.

In this chapter, I go through each imbalance and describe how it can affect your body. In chapter four, I explain how to perform simple tests on yourself to get an idea of what imbalances might be moving your chemistry in the wrong direction. Throughout the rest of the book, I go over ways to improve these imbalances and get the body moving on the right path. If people are able to help move their bodies back into a more balanced state, many of the issues or conditions that they are dealing with can often improve, or disappear altogether. I'm not suggesting that will be the case with you. I would never be that cocky in print. Every person is different. But I have seen and heard many testimonials from those who have brought about amazing results for themselves by simply learning how their specific body is operating. The body can do some astonishing things when you begin to work with it instead of against it.

Before I get into the specific imbalances, let's look at how we got here.

Hippocrates said, "Let food be your medicine. Let medicine be your food."

If we only kept it that simple. Modern medicine has gotten to where it is today, in part, through a scientific and philosophical debate that culminated in the 19th century. On one side of the debate was French microbiologist, Antoine Bechamp. On the other side was French microbiologist, Louis Pasteur. Bechamp and Pasteur strongly disagreed in their bacteriological theories and they argued heatedly about who was correct. It was kind of like watching Letterman and Oprah during their rivalry years. It was...

The Argument That Changed The Course Of Medicine

Pasteur promoted a theory of disease that described non-changeable microbes as the primary cause of disease. This is the theory of <u>monomorphism</u>. This theory says that a microorganism is static and unchangeable. It is what it is. Disease is solely caused by microbes or bacteria that invade the body from the outside. (This is also known as the germ theory.)

Bechamp held the view that microorganisms can go through different stages of development and they can evolve into various growth forms within their life cycle. This is the theory of pleomorphism. He discovered microbes in the blood that he called microzymas. These microbes would change shape as individuals became diseased and, for Bechamp, this was the cause of disease; hence, disease comes from inside the body.

Another scientist of the day, Claude Bernard, entered into the argument and said that it was actually the milieu, or the environment, that is all important to the disease process. Microbes do change and evolve, but *how* they do so is a result of the environment (or terrain) to which they are exposed. Hence, for Bernard, microbes, being pleomorphic, will change according to the environment to which they are exposed. Think of it like picking up a geeky kid, who owns every issue of *Green Lantern* comics ever printed, and dropping him off in the streets of the ghetto to see how he fairs. If that kid wants to survive, he's going to have to adapt to his surroundings. Disease in the body, as a biological process, will develop and manifest dependent upon the state of the internal biological terrain.

Both men, Bechamp and Pasteur, acknowledged certain aspects of each others' research, but it has been said that Pasteur was a stronger, more flamboyant, and a more vocal opponent to the quiet Bechamp. Pasteur also came from wealth and had influential family connections. He went to great lengths to disprove Bechamp's view. Pasteur eventually managed to convince the scientific community that his view alone was correct. Bechamp felt that this diverted science down a deplorable road—a road that held only half the truth.

The story is told that, on his deathbed, Pasteur finally acknowledged Bechamp's work as having some validity and even said, "Bernard was correct: the microbe is nothing; the terrain is everything." It was a 180-degree turnaround from his previous view. With his death imminently at hand, he as much as admitted that his germ theory had flaws. But his admission fell on deaf ears. It was far too late. It could not reverse the inertia of ideas that had already been accepted by mainstream science at that time. Allopathic (drug based) medicine was firmly entrenched on the road that was paved by Pasteur.

The result of that road is what you see today practiced as medicine. When a body is out of balance, doctors attempt to put it back into balance, first through drugs, then through surgery. The general effect is to remove the symptoms, not to deal with the ultimate cause of the ailment.

Terrain Of The Body And Biochemical Individuality

As described by Dr. Claude Bernard over one hundred years ago, of prime importance is the terrain of the body. One compartment of the body's chemistry is the interstitial fluid that bathes, nourishes and takes waste away from every cell in the human body. He believed that the imbalances in this cellular environment affected the entire body, including the immune system. Over time, a compromised immune system had difficulty fighting disease and maintaining health. This theory later developed into the science known as Biological Terrain. By looking at the environment in which our cells live, we can find strong indications about how the body is operating and uncover imbalances that may be causing trouble.

Information is truly the smallest element in our culture; every tangible item on this planet is filled with it. Today, professional science geeks can take a single hair and tell you the height, weight, sex, and race of where that hair came from because a huge amount of data lies within that hair. Everything is crammed with information. It's not information that is missing. These days it's people willing to listen to the information who are hard to find. If you look at urine and saliva, you're looking at fluids that are loaded with insight into the terrain, or environment, in which the cells are living.

Urine can provide clues about what the system is trying to throw out of the blood. Saliva is not really interstitial fluid, but it gives us an idea of what is happening in the interstitial fluid of the body. This is, more or less, what the body is holding on to. By looking at what the body is throwing out, and comparing that to what the body is holding on to, now we can start to have some discretion. When looking at markers in urine and saliva, these numbers become a mathematical reality for these fluids. You can get measurements of pH, ureas, conductivity, rH2, etc. You can get all sorts of information from urine and saliva and I explain them all in chapter four.

The information you find through looking at your chemistry is very individualized. It is like snowflakes. You will see patterns that are common, like every snowflake has six sides. However, within the patterns, the combination is never the same. We don't see two people the same. What you're looking for is to prioritize the information you find. What do I need most of all? People are so undernourished today, they often need about 2/3 of whatever is in any health food store in America. They are that nutritionally depleted and often in deep trouble. That being said, they can't just go in and graze on 2/3 of a health food store, that's just not reasonable. By looking at the chemistry of an individual, we are trying to assess what is going to do the most good out of all those items in that health food store.

The popular trend is for people to write about specific nutrients saying, "This nutrient is good for this condition," or "That nutrient should be used by everyone." The bio-individuality is so important because, sure, magnesium is good for everybody, but a "pushing dose" of magnesium for a lot of people could exacerbate an imbalance that may already be causing them trouble. By pushing dose, I mean an amount higher than you might find in a multivitamin. On the other side of this fence, we might find a lot of people who need magnesium desperately and the small amount found in a multivitamin wouldn't do much of anything for them. In this regard, the goal should be to look at your own individuality and ask, "What do I really need? What's the priority to my system?" not, "What is the most popular thing to buy?"

Those Who Paved The Way

To cheat a little bit and learn from those who worked in natural health in the past, I really like to look at doctors from the thirties and forties. This was a time when doctors were allowed to think in their practices. They could try to understand what was really going on with their patients without fear of being sued or losing their licenses. Since rules are established nowadays that foster profit instead of health, it's beneficial to learn from those who paved the way seventy or eighty years ago. Human physiology hasn't changed much in the last 100 years and my respect for the pioneers in health care will be evident throughout the book. It is specifically those named below who created the work that makes up the bulk of what I cover in this series.

For those who like to learn more, I have added more information about these brilliant minds in Appendix B, in the back of the book. When I mention Dr. Carey Reams, Dr. Emanuel Revici, Thomas Riddick, Dr. Melvin Page, or Dr. Royal Lee, you'll know you can flip to Appendix B to learn more about these early pioneers. To save space and get to the point faster, I'll skip the introductions for now and start describing the ideas we have gained from their research.

Intro To Imbalances

In chapter six I explain all the imbalances you will be learning about in this book. I first want to teach you how to test yourself and how to understand the results of those tests in chapters four and five. That way, you'll know which imbalances you need to pay close attention to. For now, I'll give you a very brief introduction to each imbalance. I mention these imbalances in the next couple chapters so I want you to be able to follow along. Each imbalance has a polar opposite so I'll go over them in pairs.

Electrolyte Excess and Electrolyte Deficiency Imbalances

These imbalances demonstrate the level of electrolytes in the system. An Electrolyte Excess Imbalance would show that there are too many minerals in the system and a possible inability for the body to remove junk, often resulting in high blood pressure. Almost 50% of Americans fall into this category.

An Electrolyte Deficiency Imbalance would show a lack of mineral in the system, leaving the body without enough resources to function properly. Many readers of this book likely fall into this category.

Anabolic and Catabolic Imbalances

These imbalances describe cellular permeability. Whether or not the body is in the breaking down or building up phase is a major focus when it comes to these two imbalances. Knowing cellular permeability can give you system-wide information instead of the tunnel vision that symptoms normally provide.

Beta Oxidizer and Tricarb Oxidizer

The body is designed to burn both glucose and fats, generally speaking. Some individuals get stuck burning more fats than glucose, or vice versa. If one of these imbalances shows as a result of your self-tests, you would likely be burning predominantly fat or glucose. This is key information for those who wish to increase their energy or lose a little weight.

Sympathetic and Parasympathetic Imbalances

The two extremes of our autonomic nervous system (described further in chapter six) are the fight or flight state or the rest and digest state. If an individual is stuck in one state or the other, health issues can arise.

Acid and Alkaline Imbalances

Okay, don't get me started just yet. For now, let's just say that these imbalances have to do with the pH of your bloodstream and leave it at that. Once I get going about these imbalances, it can be hard to shut me up. You'll see.

CHAPTER FOUR

Testing

Now comes the fun part. This book is a hands-on, roll up your sleeves and get your face dirty type of do-it-yourself guide. It's going to take some actual effort to figure out any imbalances that you might be currently experiencing. Since work will be involved, this is a great place to start weeding out those readers who would rather complain about government policies, than learn to make correct dietary choices. You can use this chapter as a great gauge for yourself. If you find yourself skipping this section, and you don't take time to find proper testing tools and run these tests on your own chemistry, the odds that you're going to be willing to make the nutritional and lifestyle changes necessary to see any results are about as good as me showing up at your house and mowing your lawn. Keep in mind that I don't know where you live and I haven't mowed a lawn since I was twelve.

Yes, you will need to do the work if you want to have the reward. However, with the Internet at hand, it's possible to get help or guidance, no matter where you are, if you choose. Acquiring this information about your own chemistry is really pretty easy. None of the tests I am about to explain will take any longer than it takes you to brush your teeth, and you do that every day, right? I don't know you, but I do feel like we have this bond, and if I have a bond with you, I really want you to be brushing your teeth at least once a day. That's just my policy. I'll tell you what, we're just going to assume that you brush your teeth. Since you know you have time for that every day, you'll be able to find time to look at your chemistry too—just make it a habit. You won't even need to test yourself every day, in most cases. Obviously, the worse off you are, the more often you will want to test yourself so you can gain more insight. But, generally speaking, most people can look at their chemistry a couple times a week while they're trying to see improvements. If you achieve the health improvements that you're looking for, you can choose to test yourself less frequently and maybe just check in periodically to see where you are.

The most exciting part about what I teach you in this chapter is this: By becoming a participant in your own health and tracking the results from your self-tests, you will be able to watch your progress and know if you're going in the right direction, even before your symptoms change. How fun is that? A tremendous number of people will try to make changes in their diet, or try something else new in order to improve an issue they are dealing with, or lose some weight, or any number of goals they are trying to reach; but when results don't show up in the first two weeks, they say, "This crap doesn't work," and they quit. Obviously, they haven't been exposed to the reality that the body is agricultural, like a crop, or a plant. The body can start getting better, but it doesn't just change in two weeks because you want it to. Changes in nature take time. If you plant watermelon seeds on Saturday, you can't come back on Thursday and say, "Hey, where the hell are my melons?" You wouldn't think, "I guess I'm just not good at growing big oval-shaped stuff." You wouldn't dig up the seeds or stomp on the sprouts and try to plant squash to see if that would work better.

We, as intelligent humans, understand that gardening involves a process under the surface of the ground and that process can take time. That seed is sprouting and that plant is pushing its way slowly to the surface. We can't see any results, but we understand that we need to be patient and let nature take its course. We don't dig up what we plant every week while the neighbors listen to us cuss at the ground yelling, "Damn, tomatoes don't work either!" If this behavior sounds ridiculous in the garden, why is it so widely accepted when it comes to our body? By using powerful and toxic drugs that are only produced to force a symptom out of existence, our society has become accustomed to a "fix me now" mentality. If your oil light comes on in the dashboard of your car and you take a screwdriver and break out the bulb so that it doesn't glow anymore, have you fixed the problem the oil light was indicating? If you want to improve your health naturally, you will need to "fix" the way you think and allow your body the time and resources it needs to create the improvements you want to see.

Think about it, anything that happens quickly with the body is usually bad. A bone snaps, a tendon tears, you get poked in the eye... these are all things that happen quickly. The "fix-me-now" mentality of the medical world is not the best route to go in most cases. I do believe there is a segment of society that is starting to understand that. There will always be people who want the quick fix, but my opinion is that the viewpoint of the public is beginning to change. After all, things do change. We used to think smoking was healthy, we used to think Earth was flat, and look at all the kids that wear helmets now when they ride their bikes. When did our heads get so soft? I know first hand that it is possible to be looking at a girl on the sidewalk and drive a bike into the back of a parked car, helmet-free, without hurting your head. We didn't wear helmets when I was growing up. When I was young, if we saw a kid wearing a helmet, we would all stop to see what he was going to do. "Wait! Let's watch this kid. He's definitely about to try something crazy, he's wearing a helmet." The only time you saw a helmet on a little dude riding a bike was when he was about to utter the phrase, "I'm gonna try something rad. I saw it on a cartoon once but I think I can do it." Now, the viewpoint on helmets has changed because stuff changes. That's just how it works. Soon enough, I believe it will be widely accepted that to improve an underlying cause of a health issue, you need to make gradual, agricultural changes in the body so the actual problem can be resolved.

Since symptoms will often take time to improve, the measurements you will be taking can become almost like x-ray vision glasses that allow you to look "beneath the soil" to verify imbalances are moving in the direction you want them to. (It's upsetting to think about how many pairs of x-ray glasses I ordered from the back of comic books as a kid. I really wanted those to work. I ended up just having to stare at *Cosmopolitan* covers at a steep angle—that didn't help either.)

As you chart your self-test numbers, you will see patterns, improvements, or maybe have the realization that you need input from a professional health coach. If your chemistry is moving in a more balanced direction, you can view that as a good indication that you're taking the proper steps toward improved health. If you feel the same or there is no change in the issues you are experiencing, but your chemistry hasn't shifted yet either, then the way you feel makes sense according to your chemistry and you may need to just do more work to get your chemistry to move. I have seen some people with severe imbalances and they can throw the whole kitchen sink into the mix and still have a hard time affecting their chemistry in the beginning. You may also be making some choices that are pushing you further toward an imbalance at the same time you are trying to correct that same imbalance. For example, eating sugar will push most people more anabolic. You could be using supplements to help push your body away from that anabolic imbalance, but if you're still cramming snack cakes in your mouth every few hours, you're going to have a hard time overpowering all that sugar.

To look at the other side of that coin, if your chemistry moves in a more balanced direction and you feel worse, don't take that lightly. I don't like to view feeling lousy as a "healing crisis." If you're feeling worse, don't look at this book like, "It's so brilliant, everything he's writing must apply directly to me." This book was not written with your chemistry in mind and at the moment, I'm not even wearing pants. I'm not sure that's a critical piece of information, but it does illustrate the point that I'm just a guy sitting at his desk, miles away from wherever you are currently located. I can't possibly know where your chemistry is if I'm not even wearing the proper clothing to present myself outdoors. Don't just read something in a book and assume it must be appropriate for you without understanding how it pertains to you and your chemistry. You may need help from someone who works in this field and understands the intricacies of how different imbalances can change how the body is operating. It can be easy to understand how any one imbalance affects the body. But if you have layer upon layer of imbalances, all affecting each other and how the body is working, that can become quite a puzzle and you may need some help. If that help happens to come from me and you work with me in person, I promise to be fully clothed.

Even when you're looking at your own chemistry instead of just your symptoms, there is no guarantee that one particular imbalance is creating the symptom you want to improve. For example, I've talked about how an Electrolyte Deficiency Imbalance can contribute to the symptom, menstrual cramps. You could have severe menstrual cramps, test yourself and see that the numbers indicate an extreme electrolyte deficiency, do the work to improve that imbalance—and still have menstrual cramp issues. How is that fair? I'm not saying that it's fair, but sometimes symptoms can have multiple underlying causes, one on top of the other. Correcting one of the underlying causes may not be enough to correct the annoying symptom. That's why it's so important to work toward bringing the body into balance instead of just trying to correct an imbalance that you think is creating the symptom you want to see go away. In chapter nine, I talk more about how to help your whole body instead of just an imbalance. For now, keep in mind the body is a complicated piece of equipment. There is often a lot more going on than any of us will ever realize. You can merely take the information that you have and use it to the best of your ability to help your own body work its magic.

If you feel worse or you get stuck, get help. If you can't afford help, keep seeking knowledge until you find the answers you're looking for. Answers are out there. Don't think that you're a lost cause. If you're dealing with an issue, somebody on this planet has corrected that issue. When I was sick, I became such a psycho researcher that I began to know more than the professionals who were trying to help me. The online university at www.CoalitionUniversity.org is filled with people who take classes just to better understand how the body works. Many of the students are not even looking to work in the field. They are simply trying to learn more to help themselves or a loved one who is dealing with health issues. They're tired of the medical world trying to help them with poisons, and they're searching for their own answers. The university even offers several free courses, so log on and see what you can learn.

Advanced Tests

Some people will be able to create life-changing improvements with very little information. Many will completely change the way they feel just by improving their digestion. Digestion is so huge I blab on and on about it for two chapters in this book. Improving digestion really helps a lot of people. Still, others will need to do a lot more work. If you fall into this category, and you don't see the improvements you would like to see, consider how much information you were able to gather about your chemistry. In Appendix A, under *Advanced Tests*, I share with you some industry secrets and explain how professionals can get a panoramic view of how a person's body is chugging through this world. I explain all the tests that can be run, the equipment that can be used, and how this information can be pieced together to get a picture of where things might be going awry.

This is what you really want. You really want this full picture and all the data that can be seen in this "snapshot." But the snapshot costs money, either by paying for the professional's help or by buying your own equipment and taking the courses required to learn how to use it. Many of these courses can be completed online and the equipment is affordable enough that many people buy it just for their own personal use since it can be a lot less expensive than a year's prescription of just about any drug. Be sure to understand, however, that buying some equipment and taking some courses does not mean that you can diagnose your own illnesses or prescribe medications to your neighbor who helps you put up your Christmas lights every year. Diagnosing and prescribing are things that are done by medical doctors in the medical world.

This work is about understanding your specific body, how it is operating, and the nutrition and lifestyle changes that might make you feel better. It's not about diagnosing or treating. Those are words that are used in the medical world and we don't use those here. Even if you work with a natural health professional, you're just being educated about your body and about health and nutrition so you can make your own informed decisions. Nobody is going to hand you a bottle of pills and you will be all better. You're still going to have to do the work, make the choices, and take the responsibility. At least, in this scenario, you will understand why you are doing that work.

I put the information about advanced testing at the end of the book so you will have a foundation of knowledge under your belt before we cover those tests. Since not everyone can afford professional help or testing equipment, I'm going to start by breaking down some much less expensive testing tools you can pick up at just about any health food store and/or pharmacy. These tools will give you a smaller picture, but for a lot of readers, it will be enough to give you an idea of what is going on. I feel it's important to show you the real deal, let you see how professionals are doing this work and then leave it up to you to decide how much of the picture you want to see. I set up three levels of testing (with the *Advanced Tests* found in Appendix A) so you can figure out which one fits best in your life. You can try the cheap and easy level and if you are able to get the results you want, more power to you. If not, you may need to step up to the next level. Think of it like wearing a fanny pack. Yes, you want the convenience of having all your belongings on your person without having to carry them, but you also don't want to look like the idiot who is wearing a fanny pack. First, you just buy one but decide it's too embarrassing to wear. Then you think, "I'm just running to the store real quick; nobody will see me," so you take it to the next level. Pretty soon you're wearing three packs at once and everyone is calling you "fanny boy." In any case, you will need to figure out what level is appropriate for you.

Let's Get To Testing...

If you haven't acquired the necessary testing materials that I talked about at the end of chapter one, are you procrastinating, or are you just a really fast reader? Now is the time to have those tools so you can see where your chemistry is before I talk more about each imbalance. It's easy to listen to symptoms that go along with each imbalance and say, "Oh yeah, that's totally me, I must have that imbalance." But that's the wrong way to look at your individuality.

Let's say that you desperately need to go to Hallmark to pick up a card from their "I accidentally called my mother-in-law fat" section. When you get to the mall, the first thing you look for is the directory. Once you find Hallmark on the directory, what do you do next? That's right, you look for the "You Are Here" red dot. If you don't know where you are, how are you going to find where you need to go? Testing is finding the red dot.

To get the ball rolling, I will break the tests into the following sections:

- Simple Frequently Used Tests
- Intermittent Tests
- Bonus Tests
- Advanced Tests (In Appendix A)

Some of you may not need to run all of these tests. Many of you will be able to run just a few procedures and the results will be so clear, it will give you an obvious path to follow. Others will need to use more tests, and some readers will need to seek the help of a professional who can look at other parameters of their chemistry. Many of these professionals have special equipment or software that can supply information about your chemistry beyond the methods I provide in this book.

In this section you will find a *Data Tracking Sheet*. You can also go to www.KickItInTheNuts.com and download a free pdf to print so you'll be able to see the colors on the *Urine Test Strip* chart and you won't have to mark up your pretty book. This will allow you to keep a binder of your progress so you can track your results and see patterns. You will also have that information available in case you decide to seek help from a professional. Click on the link BOOK TOOLS to download the *Data Tracking Sheet*. You will need to register on the site for free to access BOOK TOOLS, as I only make these tools available to those who have read one of my books. The registration form will ask you for a "Top Secret Book Reader Code." Use: "skedaddle" in the secret code box to complete your registration and download your *Data Tracking Sheet*. While you're there, you can also download the *Imbalance Guide* and I will explain that form in the following chapter.

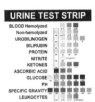

Date _____ Time _____	Date _____ Time _____	Date _____ Time _____	Date _____ Time _____
Well-Being _____	Well-Being _____	Well-Being _____	Well-Being _____

Water Intake _____

Urine pH _____

Saliva pH _____

Breath Rate _____

Breath Hold _____

Resting Standing

Blood Pressure (Systolic) _____ _____

Blood Pressure (Diastolic) _____ _____

Pulse _____ _____

You can go to www.KickItInTheNuts.com and download a free color pdf to print so you don't have to mark up your pretty book, and you'll be able to see the colors on the *Urine Test Strip* chart.

70

The Coalition

There is an international association called *The Coalition for Health Education*. This private, nonprofit association spans the planet and consists of doctors, health coaches, nutritionists, a wide variety of other types of natural health professionals and members of the general public who want to learn more about natural health and how the body really works. When readers come to www.KickItInTheNuts.com looking for a health coach who can help them better understand the ideas that are taught in this book, we send them to *The Coalition* to find a professional in their area.

We have also made arrangements with this private association to allow our readers to become members without sponsorship from a professional health coach. *The Coalition* has an advanced website that was put in place to help health coaches educate their clients and monitor the progress of their client's chemistry. As those clients input the numbers from their self-tests into the website, the health coach can help them make adjustments according to their chemistry. However, even if you are not working with a health coach, as one of my readers, you can register as a member of the site, which will grant you access to all of your own advanced monitoring and tracking tools. I helped them put together many of the systems they use today so they have given my readers the hook-up. As you input the results of your self-tests into the system, you can watch the changes over time in the site's dynamic graphing systems. You can even keep a food journal to which your self-test results will transfer automatically so you can see how different foods affect your chemistry and how you feel. You will also find charts that can show you where your chemistry is now, and what foods can help push you in the right direction if you are imbalanced.

It is an amazing tool. The best part is that $20 per year will cover your membership dues and there is no extra charge to use the tools on the website. As an added benefit, if you decide that you need the help of a professional in your area, *The Coalition* can attach your account to a local health coach who can then see how your chemistry has been moving while you were working on your own.

The *Data Tracking Sheet*, that you can download on the KickItInTheNuts.com website, is an adequate way to keep tabs on your chemistry; but if you really want to see the whole picture by using the graphs and other tools, *The Coalition* is the way to go. If you have an Internet connection and can afford $20 for the year, you'll want to take advantage of this arrangement. It has been a very helpful tool for the *Kick It in the Nuts* readers. For the remainder of this book, it may sound like I'm assuming you are using the tools on *The Coalition* website because I feel like they can really help you see into your numbers and better understand your chemistry. I assume that you are using them because they are helpful tools that will make this process much easier. You can call me lazy if you like, but I tend to move toward methods that make my life easier.

Investing in your own health is as important as taking the time to read about it. Though improving the actual cause of a problem can take work and sometimes money, I always tell my clients that sooner or later you're going to pay for your health. You can pay now and the money you spend will go toward preventative measures and long term improvement, or you can pay later and those funds will go toward holding you together or trying to repair something that has gone horribly wrong. We all pay, the option of <u>when</u> is up to us.

If you ignore your health long enough it'll go away.

You can learn more on our website, www.KickItInTheNuts.com, or go directly to www.OurCoaltion.org and click on Self-Monitoring Registration.

Testing Procedures

Here they come...

Frequently Used Tests

It can be helpful to perform these evaluations on a regular basis, at least in the beginning. They are very simple and can easily fit into your current daily activities once you make them a habit. I like to see people run most of these tests at least twice a week for the first few weeks so you can get an idea of where your chemistry truly is. This becomes the "You Are Here" dot on the mall directory.

pH of Urine and Saliva

It is best if you don't test your urine pH right when you wake up. The first morning urine test, while being a valid test, takes greater discretion to sort out the results because you are unloading the previous day's "metabolic debt," those acids you accumulated through the previous day. Understanding the results of that first morning test is quite complicated and I don't cover that in this book. Testing your urine and saliva pH either just before lunch or just before dinner (ideally at least two hours since you have eaten any food) will be an easier test to discern what the numbers are showing.

Urine pH: Simply hold the test strip in your urine stream for a second and read against the color chart. If the chart reads in half-point increments, and your reading is between two colors, make an estimate for your reading. For example, if the color on your pH strip falls between 6 and 6.5, make a guess and say 6.3 or wherever you think it lands. Just pick a number and don't say "really green" or "very yellow," because that is too subjective. Pick a number; you are simply looking for a range. If the actual reading is off by a little bit, that's okay. You won't be using NASA equipment here and you're not going to get an exact reading. You just want to be able to see, "Is it high or is it low? How high or low is it?" So, don't drive yourself nuts and think that you have to pull out the magnifying glass and read the strip under indoor lighting that mimics the sun at high noon. Just look at the pee on the strip and mark it down.

Saliva pH: Try not to drink or have anything in your mouth for 20 minutes before testing, and ideally you want to wait at least two hours after eating. Testing your saliva at the same time as your urine will keep everything simple. Don't use the same strip for both—it makes me sad that I feel like I need to explain that (however I do know one person who takes a pair of scissors and splits the strip long ways to get twice as many measurements out of a pack). Bring up a little saliva between your lips and run the test strip across your lips and through the saliva. Read against the chart right away. Timing is important. The CO_2 in your saliva will out-gas into the atmosphere. The reading will often rise the longer you wait to read it. Because of this, it is best to read the saliva as soon as you moisten the strip or you will have a less accurate reading. With urine, it is not as important to read against the chart right away.

Blood Pressure

To test your resting blood pressure, lie down and relax for two minutes or so. Perform the test on your left arm according to the directions for your blood pressure cuff. If you are using an automatic cuff, it will likely display three numbers, usually in this configuration: The top number is the systolic pressure (measure of blood pressure while the heart is beating). The middle number is the diastolic pressure (measure of blood pressure while the heart is relaxed). The bottom number will be your pulse. If it is hard for you to lie down for the reading, you can take this test in a seated, resting position. I include another blood pressure test you can do under the intermittent tests section.

Breath Rate

This can be difficult to test on yourself. When you're conscious of what you're doing, you might adjust your breathing, even subconsciously. Anytime you can, get someone else to test this for you so you can let your mind wander to other things and just breathe normally. Doing so will likely provide a more accurate reading. If you don't have that option, just try to count your breaths while breathing as normally as possible. Lie down and relax. Try to think of other things so that you breathe normally. Start your timer and count the number of times you inhale in 30 seconds. Double that number for the amount of breaths per minute. Just be sure you don't count an inhale as one and an exhale as two. Only count the inhales. I like to continue for the entire minute to see if I get the same number the last 30 seconds as I did the first. If not, I may average the two. My preference is to use an egg timer, so you can set it for one minute and the timer will count down to zero, allowing you to count your inhales without having to worry about the timer since it will beep when the minute is up. This can be the easiest way to perform this test if you don't have someone to help you.

Breath Hold Time

Sit comfortably. Take three full, deep breaths in and out. Near the end of the fourth inhale, start your stopwatch or timer and hold your breath as long as you can. Don't pass out or turn blue or make this like it's a contest you have to win. Guys will typically try to hold their breath longer, as if this is some type of macho sign. Not once have I noticed a girl across a room, walked up to her and said, "Hey, watch how long I can hold my breath." So guys, just know that this is not as cool as you may think it to be. That being said, do hold your breath as long as you comfortably can. It's best not to look at the stopwatch while you're holding your breath. If you do, you may be inclined to turn it into a competition and hold your breath longer than you normally would.

75

Intermittent Tests

These are great tests that everyone should run initially, if you have the ability to do so. You won't need to run most of these tests as often as you may the frequently used tests, but they can still provide excellent information as you get started. I have placed the blood glucose test in this section because most people won't need to check this frequently. However, if you test your fasting blood sugar (first thing in the morning before you eat or drink anything other than water) and it is 100 or higher, you should make sure to acquire your own glucometer and test this nearly every day until you have your fasting blood glucose in a better range. I really like to see between 80-95. If your blood sugar is higher than 105, I recommend reading *Kick Type II Diabetes in the Nuts* as soon as it becomes available. I'm not saying that you have Diabetes if your blood sugar is over 105, but the guidelines laid out in that book can help you get your fasting blood sugar down to an acceptable range.

I encourage you not to skip this initial blood glucose test, even if you've recently had your blood tested by your doctor and he or she said the glucose levels were "okay." It's best to work off of the actual number. Most people reading this book will have their fasting blood sugar show up in a good range. But if your sugars are high, and you don't know it, you could work for a long time trying to correct other areas with little result because the high sugars can make some issues much harder to improve.

Blood Glucose

Wash your hands prior to testing so residues from lotions, etc. don't affect the test results. Insert a new disposable lancet into your lancing device. (Never re-use lancets. You may also be using an all-in-one disposable lancet where you just remove the plastic safety cover from the needle, cock the lancet and push a button to set it off while holding the tip to your finger.) Prick your finger and allow the blood to make a small bubble. (It's best not to squeeze your finger, if you can avoid doing so, since that may give you a lower blood sugar reading.) Depending on your glucometer, either drip the blood on top of the test strip or place the test strip up against the drop of blood and it will sip the blood up into the strip like a straw. To get your fasting glucose, test before breakfast, before you drink anything other than water, and, if possible, before you brush your teeth. When you want to check your fasting glucose, it's best to leave the glucometer out where you will see it first thing in the morning so you won't forget.

Resting to Standing - Blood Pressure Test

To get an indication of how your body is recovering from a given stress, you can perform a "resting to standing" blood pressure reading. You will actually take your blood pressure reading two times in a row during this test.

#1 - To test your resting blood pressure: Lie down and test on your left arm according to the directions for your blood pressure cuff, just like you did previously in your normal resting blood pressure test.

#2 - To test your standing blood pressure: Remain in a lying position, push the button to start the inflation again, then stand up and hold your arm still as not to disturb the machine from taking its reading. You may need to have the machine in your other hand so you can hold it as still as possible as you get up. If the tube from the cuff to the machine is long enough, setting the machine on a table next to you is the best option. If the tube is not long enough, you will have to try to hold the machine as still as possible (along with holding yourself as still as possible) so the machine will not show an error code and require you to retest. If you do get an error code, you will want to lie back down for about 30 seconds to relax and do both steps one and two again.

Since you won't likely perform this test very often, a space is not reserved for it on the *Data Tracking Sheet*. Instead, just place both resting and standing readings on each line separated by a slash.

For example, your systolic pressure line might look like this: 122/130. The 122 would indicate your systolic (top) number while you were lying down and the 130 would represent your systolic number when you were standing up. Then, you can do the same thing for your diastolic and pulse numbers. The ideal result is to see your standing systolic reading higher than your resting systolic reading. If the standing number is lower, this can be an indication that the system may be having a hard time recovering from a given stress.

Dermographic Line

To perform this test, run the non-ink side of a pen across the inside of your arm and then wait 20-30 seconds to see if your skin turns red, white, or the mark just disappears. If the mark disappears, you would be considered balanced in this test.

This is an autonomic nervous system indicator. Typically if a person's vascular system is constricted, the dermographic line stays with a white center and can indicate the individual is leaning too far on the sympathetic side. If the dermographic line stays red, that can indicate a person is leaning toward the parasympathetic side.

Gag Reflex

Gag reflex is another indicator of the autonomic nervous system. High gag reflex is indicating that a person is leaning toward the parasympathetic side. The lack of a gag reflex indicates a leaning toward the sympathetic side. No test is required here. Simply ask yourself, if I'm brushing my teeth and the toothbrush goes a little too far back, do I gag?

Pupil Size

Pupil size is another indicator of the autonomic nervous system. Small pupils indicate parasympathetic; large pupils indicate sympathetic. Looking at the colored area of your eye, if your pupils cover less than 25% of that space, they can be considered small. If your pupils cover more than 50% of the colored area, they can be considered large. If your pupils take up between 25% - 50% of the colored space, this can be considered normal.

11-Parameter Urine Dipstick

On the website, www.NaturalReference.com, you can find a product, Urispec 11-way urine test strips. A canister of 100 test strips will run you about $45 and very few people will need to order these more than once. These strips are an excellent tool to give you insights that you would normally learn only by visiting a health professional. The Urispec 11-way urine test strips (also referred to as a 10-parameter urine test strip) measure blood, urobilinogen, bilirubin, protein, nitrite, ketones, ascorbic acid, glucose, pH, specific gravity and leukocytes. Not only can these measurements help you recognize which imbalances may be the most severe for you, but also, individuals could uncover some fairly major issues that could cause all kinds of trouble if undetected. In my opinion, with these test strips, people can uncover information that may be more valuable to their health than anything they would find in most traditional blood tests—all for about forty five cents a strip.

When using an 11-parameter urine test strip, all of the measurements can be read right away except the leukocytes reading. You want to start a two-minute egg timer as soon as you dampen the test strip and read the leukocytes box right at that two minute time. Pee into a cup and then dip the strip all the way into the cup. You may have to bend the strip a little by pushing the strip against the bottom of the cup in order to get all the colored boxes covered in urine. Pull the strip out right away and tap its edge on a paper towel to wick away some of the excess urine. Read the colors against the color chart on the strips container. On the *Data Tracking Sheet*, circle the colored boxes that match the colors on your dipstick for each reading.

This dipstick is a great, cheap way to look at some more in-depth numbers. I recommend using this 11-parameter dipstick at least once to get a bigger picture of what is going on with your body. For those who would like to learn more about the parameters covered on these strips, I have provided more detailed explanations in Appendix A. Some of the words are all big and fancy. You don't really need to understand them right now. I just want to let you know what's available on these dipsticks. In this section, I give you a quick blurb about some of these variables. I don't spend time defining what some of these terms mean. Instead, I just let you know what indications they can provide and you can dig into Appendix A if you're still keen for more.

- Non-Hemolyzed / Hemolyzed
Blood should not be seen in urine. If it is, that could be an indication of either kidney or bladder distress or trauma. Sometimes non-hemolyzed blood can be seen during a woman's monthly cycle; if that is the case, the test should be administered again at a different time of the month.

- Bilirubin
Bilirubin should not be seen in the urine. When bilirubin is seen in the urine, that means it did not go out the biliary pathway, down through the intestines and out the south gate (your butt). It is a validator that the biliary pathway isn't running as nicely as it should. Since bile flow is so important for digestion and waste removal, this is an excellent parameter to have access to.

- Urobilinogen
Urobilinogen is not normally seen in urine. Urobilinogen is bilirubin that has been eaten for lunch in the intestines by bacteria. When bacteria eats bilirubin, they poop urobilinogen. This can be common if an individual is constipated.

• Protein

Protein should not be seen in the urine. If it is, that can be an indicator that the kidneys may be overwhelmed. Protein in the urine can also be an indicator that the body is breaking down its own tissue.

• Nitrite

A positive reading for nitrite is one of the indicators of a UTI (urinary tract infection)—some type of bacteria in the bladder.

• Ketones

Ketones are produced by the burning of fat. Typically diabetics show ketones because they are not burning carbohydrates, they are burning fat. People on the Atkins Diet were given ketone strips to show that they had reached the goal of ketosis, so that they would burn fat. I'm not saying this is your goal. This parameter can help you understand if your body is predisposed to burn more fat or more glucose.

• Ascorbic Acid

Ascorbic acid will alter the readings on the dipstick. So while this reading lets you know how much ascorbic acid might be being excreted in the urine, it also alerts you that some of the reagents may react improperly when there is too much ascorbic acid.

• Glucose

The dipstick color chart shows that some glucose in the urine is "normal." I might agree that is "common" however one would not want to conclude that it is optimal or "normal." I don't think it is correct that glucose should be in people's urine. Typically you see a glucose reading in the negative box, showing no glucose—that is how you want to see it.

• pH

I already talked about pH in the simple tests section. This is just nice to have on the strip so you can conveniently check pH with all the other parameters.

• Specific Gravity

Specific gravity can be used to validate whether or not your body is leaning too anabolic or too catabolic. This alone is not an indication, however, it can be a great piece of data when looking for further confirmation.

• Leukocytes

If you see both leukocytes and nitrite in the urine, that is a very positive indicator of a urinary tract infection and bacteria in the bladder.

I talk more about what to look for with your dipstick results when I cover *Understanding Your Imbalances* in chapter five.

Bonus Tests

Spit Test

Before going to bed, place a clear glass full of water on your bathroom counter or wherever you go first thing in the morning when you wake up. Seeing the glass will help remind you to do this test—so you don't brush your teeth first. Make sure the glass is transparent so you can see what's going on inside. Immediately upon waking, swallow the saliva in your mouth and bring up new saliva. Let it drop gently into the glass on top of the water. Now watch what happens. You're looking to see if the saliva floats on top of the water or if it starts to string down into the water. Watch for approximately thirty seconds. If it strings down, note how quickly it happens. If it strings down into the glass a lot, that can be an indication of an infection.

A lack of iron can be a contributing factor to menstrual cramps for some women. My thought is that if a woman has low· iron, it's most commonly because she is vegetarian/vegan or because her digestion is not working well enough to pull the iron out of the food she is eating. Poor digestion is the more frequent cause, believe it or not. With this in mind, I feel that if people take the proper steps to correct their digestion, iron will come back into the system in the proper amounts. I talk in depth about digestion in chapter seven.

If you <u>know</u> that your iron levels are low and you think this could be contributing to your cramps, you may be able to get some faster relief by supplementing a good source of iron, like concentrated cherry juice. However, you really need to know where your iron levels are before you start using iron supplements. Even though women who still get their period regularly have a much lower risk, the dangers of iron overload are more common than you may think and are rarely discovered in the medical world.

Hemochromatosis

Hemochromatosis is also known as iron overload. Women who still get their period regularly have a much lower risk of experiencing any iron overload conditions since you bleed out iron every month. All the same, since excessive iron levels can cause so much trouble, it's really smart to know your iron levels before you start to use any iron supplements. You can find out for free by donating blood. When you donate blood to the Red Cross, they will always check your iron levels first to make sure you can afford to give up any iron before they start draining blood out of your arm like a giant mosquito. If your iron is too low, they won't let you donate. They will prick your finger and put a drop of your blood into a little box that will output a number indicating your blood iron levels. Below 12.5, they won't let you donate. It is not likely that your number will exceed 15; but if it does, you may want to have a full iron panel done at a lab. I will provide you with a website where you can order one through the Internet, without · a doctor's prescription, since it is used only for educational purposes.

There is a hereditary DNA malfunction, hemochromatosis, which is very common for men of Irish or Scottish descent. I am both Irish and Scottish, yet 23 doctors never figured out that I have hemochromatosis. Even though my iron levels were through the roof, nobody picked up on it. One doctor even asked me if I eat a lot of spinach. I told him no and he simply said, "Good, don't." That was it. Seeing that there is no drug or expensive procedure to correct hemochromatosis, it simply isn't in a doctor's ongoing education, since that education is most commonly provided by pharmaceutical companies.

For this book, the majority of readers will very likely have more low-iron issues than iron-overload issues. I simply want to add this information to all of our titles to spread awareness of this problem, especially for males (or females who no longer have a period) who are of Irish or Scottish descent. The medical world has removed the iron panel from most standard blood tests to cut down on costs, but they will add it on your test for free if you ask. You just have to know to ask. This condition is very easily treated if you know it is a problem for you. If you don't know, it can certainly cause a world of trouble and baffle doctor after doctor, run up a six figure medical bill, and flat out be annoying.

In the past, I have used the website www.HealthCheckUSA.com to order iron panels without a doctor's prescription. You simply buy the test online (it will run you about $60) and they email you a form to take into the lab. You just show up with the form and they draw a blood sample. You'll get your results back in a week or two. You may need a professional to help you interpret them, but the result sheet usually at least indicates if specific numbers are high or low. If your numbers are high, the same website also has a hemochromatosis DNA test you can order to find out if you carry any hemochromatosis genes.

It's all about education. There is now a wide variety of tests that you can order online in this manner. It's very easy to do and most tests are reasonably priced. It really works just like when your doctor sends you to a lab for a test, but in this scenario, the test results are sent to the online company and they send you a copy too (either by mail or email). There is value in consumers having the ability to learn about their own bodies so there are companies that can make this happen without a doctor.

CHAPTER FIVE

Understanding Your Imbalances

The previous chapter showed you how to run simple tests to help you see your biological identity. The next step is for me to help you understand how these numbers can be translated into imbalances. In other words, now we can look at how whacked you really are. Most people live their life by monitoring symptoms. But occasionally, by the time symptoms show up, these people are in real trouble. So, I'm going to teach you how to know when some symptoms could be coming, before they even get there. In this way, instead of reacting to symptoms, you can become proactive through measurement. Even though one of the goals of this book is to sway you from living your life through symptoms, you can still use symptoms to further understand where your body chemistry may be going awry. Symptoms become more meaningful when they are seen in a context of biological measurement.

In chapter four I showed you the *Data Tracking Sheet* I created to help you monitor changes in your chemistry. Later in this chapter, I explain how to use the far superior tools on *The Coalition* website; but for now, printing off one of these *Data Tracking Sheets* is a great way to get started. You can download the pdf from our website, www.KickItInTheNuts.com. Just click on BOOK TOOLS and DATA TRACKING SHEET. (Don't forget you need to register for free as described in chapter four, and download your *Imbalance Guide* while you're at it.)

On the tracking sheet, there are data boxes for twelve different testings. Each time you test yourself, just add the date and time to the top of one of the boxes and input your numbers. You see spaces for water intake, urine pH, saliva pH, breath rate and breath hold. We left a blank space below breath hold for those who may need to check their fasting glucose daily. Below breath hold you can input your blood pressure reading, which will include your systolic blood pressure (the top number), diastolic blood pressure (the number below the systolic), and your pulse (the very bottom number on most automatic blood pressure cuffs). In the top right corner you see a section containing colored boxes that correspond with those found on the 11-parameter urine test strips. This is where you will record the results from those strips, if you are using them. It's okay if you're not using them; the other readings will still provide valuable information. For those who need, or wish, to dig deeper into their chemistry and uncover more information, the 11-parameter urine test strips are an excellent way to go if you are not yet using a professional health coach. Since most readers won't use the 11-parameter test strips very often, we only put one block at the top of the page.

The water intake space on the *Data Tracking Sheet* should be filled in according to how much water you have had up to the point of testing for that day. This information can be useful in helping you understand why your numbers are where they are. If your blood pressure is much lower than normal, you may be able to see that you have consumed more water than normal on that day, which has brought down your blood pressure. In any case, viewing your numbers in relation to your water intake can be helpful.

I like to see people use the 11-parameter urine test strips for at least their initial test. Most people don't use these strips as often as they check their urine pH and saliva pH or blood pressure, so you might not fill in these boxes each time you input new numbers. Depending on the issues you are trying to improve, you might check only your blood pressure, breath rate, or pHs for some tests. That is acceptable and any information is helpful, in my book. (Wait a minute; this is my book, so I guess that goes without saying.) In any case, always put the date and time at the top of each box and fill in test results from that time only. It's okay to leave blanks when you don't run all of the tests. When you use the tracking tools on *The Coalition* website, you will also have the option to input only one test at time if that is all you run on a specific day.

Understanding The Data

In this chapter I cover how to look at the data from your self-tests, along with information from your life, and begin to see a picture of any imbalances that your body may be experiencing. Before we get into this, I really, really, really want to stress an important aspect of this work that I don't want you to overlook. It's pretty easy to pick up just about any book on just about any symptom, condition, infection, or whatever, read about all the symptoms and circumstances that go along with that issue, and say, "Oh yeah, that's totally me. I must have *cram pencils in my ear syndrome*," or whatever topic you are reading about. **Don't do that. It's so easy to get sucked in and believe that you have some horrific disease or condition just because the symptoms sound like something that you've experienced. Avoid doing that here while I go through the imbalances.**

I am about to cover how symptoms can be used as a piece of data, but that DOES NOT mean that the symptoms are the data. If you and I were standing in my kitchen talking about this right now, I would shake you just to make sure you were listening to me. I also really like to shake people while I try to make a funny point just to see if I can get away with it. I have a very limited number of people punch me in the neck when I do that, so it's always fun to see what I can get away with. In any case, pretend I just shook you so that the point about symptoms and jumping to conclusions sinks in.

I provide you with an *Imbalance Guide* that will let you sort the data and specific circumstances of your life all onto one page. This page will allow you to see the areas that appear to be the most imbalanced. You might say, "But this area here is sort of split. It's hard to figure out which direction this imbalance is moving." That's great. This can often be a sign of appropriate balance in this particular area. Some people might see an imbalance in each section that is covered, while others won't really see any at all. Some may see a slight imbalance that could use a little work while others may wonder how they are not falling over every time they get out of bed in the morning. Every person is different.

You're not going for a high score here. You're just trying to get a picture of how your body is operating, how you're processing food, and if there are any areas that could use a little attention. That's it. Let the picture of the *Imbalance Guide* point you in the right direction. Don't jump to the conclusion that you need to work on an imbalance because the symptoms that often go along with that imbalance are symptoms that are showing up for you. Remember, one symptom can often be created by more than one type of imbalance, or a combination of imbalances. Have you already forgotten how I shook you in my kitchen?

How Symptoms Can Help

Yes, I know I've been getting on you most of this book about how to look at your chemistry and work with the underlying causes that show up instead of trying to treat your symptoms. All of that still holds true here. What I talk about here is how to use those symptoms as another layer of data.

The more data you have, the more educated of a guess you can make about what your body chemistry snapshot looks like. If the

89

numbers for one section of the *Imbalance Guide* are leaning in one direction, but it's a little up in the air as to how severe that imbalance is, symptoms can be used as extra data to push your thinking one way or another.

For example, insomnia is a symptom that can be caused by a Catabolic Imbalance, but it can also be caused by an Electrolyte Deficiency Imbalance for completely different reasons. Insomnia can even be caused by a Sympathetic Imbalance. I will go over all of this in great detail in my upcoming book, *Kick Insomnia in the Nuts*, but my point here is that you can't pick an imbalance by a symptom since that one symptom can be created by multiple underlying causes. However, if I'm a person who deals with a lot of insomnia, and my *Imbalance Guide* showed that my numbers were leaning toward a Catabolic Imbalance, and showed no sign of an Electrolyte Deficiency Imbalance or a Sympathetic Imbalance, then I could add that insomnia piece of "data" to my *Imbalance Guide* and it may solidify the picture even more. The insomnia piece of data could now make it obvious to me that working on that Catabolic Imbalance might improve my sleep.

Again, I'm not saying that correcting a Catabolic Imbalance will "cure" insomnia. If that's what you got, you're not paying attention and you should stop and do fifteen push-ups before you go back and read that again. (F*@kin' Tony!) I'm simply saying that, if a symptom you're experiencing matches up with an imbalance that showed up in your numbers, helping that imbalance could be a great way to put your body back into a position where it can allow the whole system to operate in a healthier manner. Since sleeping is a healthy thing to do, don't you think your sleep could improve?

On the *Imbalance Guide*, under each section, you see lists of measurement ranges for some of the tests, and you may also see symptoms listed. As you check off the ranges and symptoms that apply to you, you will start to see the picture unfold. You may see the same symptom under more than one imbalance. That's okay since you understand that the same symptom can be caused by different imbalances. You dig? The following is a copy of the *Imbalance Guide*, but if you want to follow along without flipping pages back and forth, you can download the pdf from our website, www.KickItInTheNuts.com. Just click on BOOK TOOLS and IMBALANCE GUIDE. But I'm going to say it again here, just to see if I can get you to actually tell me to shut up out loud while you're reading this book in a coffee shop. Don't treat your symptoms. Just use them as additional pieces of information to guide the direction you take.

IMBALANCE GUIDE

Name: _____   Date: _____   Time: _____

ELECTROLYTE STATUS

Electrolyte Deficiency	Electrolyte Excess
Resting Systolic BP < 112 ___	___ Resting Systolic BP > 130
Standing Diastalolic BP < 73 ___	___ Standing Diastalolic BP > 87
Pulse < 70 ___	___ Hypertension
Depression ___	___ Cardiovascular Disease
Vertigo ___	___ Poor Circulation
Fatigue ___	
Insomnia ___	
Cravings ___	
Cramps ___	

CIRCADIAN RHYTHM
(CELLULAR PERMEABILITY)

Anabolic	Catabolic
Urine pH > 6.3 ___	___ Urine pH < 6.1
Saliva pH < 6.6 ___	___ Saliva pH > 6.9
Specific Gravity < 1.011 ___	___ Specific Gravity > 1.020
High Body Temp ___	___ Low Body Temp
Polyuria ___	___ Oliguria
Hard Stool / Constipation ___	___ Soft/Loose Stool
Difficult to Rise ___	___ Wake Easily
Low Debris in Urine ___	___ High Debris in Urine
Adj. Surface Tension > 69 ___	___ Adj. Surface Tension < 67
Saliva mS < 4.5 ___	___ Saliva mS > 5.5
Urine rH2 high ___	___ Urine rH2 low
Anxiety ___	___ Insomnia
	___ Slow to Heal
	___ Migraines
	___ Muscle Loss
	___ Protein on Dipstick

ENERGY PRODUCTION

Carb Burning	Fat Burning
Breath Rate > 16bpm ___	___ Breath Hold < 15bpm
Breath Hold < 50sec ___	___ Breath Hold > 50sec
Resting Systolic BP < 112 ___	___ Resting Systolic BP > 133
Glucose < 70 ___	___ Glucose > 100
Urine pH > 6.3 ___	___ Urine pH < 6.1
Saliva pH < 6.6 ___	___ Saliva pH > 6.9
Fatigue ___	___ Fatigue
Weight Issues ___	___ Weight Issues
Depression ___	___ Depression
Irritable When Hungry ___	___ Type II Diabetes

AUTONOMIC NERVOUS SYSTEM

Parasympathetic	Sympathetic
Small Pupils ___	___ Large Pupils
Pulse Pressure < 37 ___	___ Pulse Pressure > 46
Gag Reflex Increased ___	___ Gag Reflex Decreased
Red Dermographic Line ___	___ White Dermographic Line
Low Body Temp ___	___ High Body Temp
Warm Dry Hands ___	___ Cold Hands
Fingertips Warmer Than Triceps ___	___ Fingertips Colder Than Triceps
Asthma ___	___ Dry Mouth
Allergies ___	___ Food Allergies

ACID / ALKALINE BALANCE

Tending to Acidosis	Tending to Alkalosis
Breath Rate > 18bpm ___	___ Breath Rate < 14bpm
Breath Hold < 41sec ___	___ Breath Hold > 64sec
Shortness of Breath ___	___ Chronic Fatigue
	___ Sleep Apnea

DIGESTIVE ISSUES

___ Resting Systolic Blood Pressure < 112
___ Standing Diastalolic Blood Pressure < 73
___ Burping or Bloating
___ Passing Gas
___ Reflux/Heartburn
___ Total Ureas < 13
___ Light Colored Stool
___ Constipation
___ Urgent Diarrhea
___ Nausea
___ rH2 > 20 or rH2 < 17.5
___ Bilirubin on Dipstick

Electrolyte Deficiency / Electrolyte Excess
Anabolic / Catabolic
Carb Burning / Fat Burning
Parasympathetic / Sympathetic
Tending to Acidosis / Tending to Alkalosis

Again, if you don't want to mark up your pretty book,
download the pdf from our website:
www.KickItInTheNuts.com

92

Sorting Out The Data

Here is where you're going to separate yourself from all the schmucks out there who are just treating their own symptoms. Now, you're going to begin to really educate yourself on how your body is operating and areas that could use some improvement. On the *Imbalance Guide*, you see that some items have special symbols next to them. The items with a dagger symbol (†) are measurements that you will need to use the 11-parameter urine dipsticks to acquire. The delta symbol (Δ) indicates measurements acquired with use of a special set of equipment or with help from a professional. You can see that you can gain quite a lot of info with just the basic tests that were outlined in chapter four, using tools like pH strips, a blood pressure cuff, and a stop watch or egg timer.

You can follow along as I go through each measurement on the *Imbalance Guide*. Many measurements are self-explanatory, but there are a few that I describe in a little more detail because they could use extra clarification. You can then use this as a reference tool as you're filling out your *Imbalance Guide*. You don't want to check off an item if you don't really understand what it means. Having blank items is normal and should be expected. This is not like *Mad Libs* where you can just use "socks" for every noun and "dirty" for every adjective and it will work out. You want to check off only the items that are clearly a problem for you. For example, under catabolic, you see "Soft/Loose Stool." Check it off only if that is something you have been experiencing frequently, over the last month or so. Don't just check it off because you went to Mexico once and had some ass soup for two weeks. In that same regard, don't say you're not constipated if you're using two tablespoons of Milk of Magnesia every day in order to see any movement. Check off only the things that are apparent for you regularly so you don't sway your "snapshot" and make yourself look like someone you're not.

Imbalance Guide Content

Symbols Key

< less than (i.e. Pulse < 70 means Pulse is less than 70)
> greater than (i.e. Glucose > 100 means Glucose is greater than 100)
† requires a 11-parameter urine dipsticks
Δ requires special equipment or a professional

Electrolyte Status

For both of these imbalances under "Electrolyte Status," the numbers are pretty self-explanatory. *Resting Systolic BP* is the top number of your blood pressure while you are lying down or resting in a seated position. *Standing Diastolic BP* is the bottom number of your blood pressure while you are in a standing position (this is the middle number if you are using an automated machine that also measures pulse). *Pulse* is the number that comes up on the very bottom of most automatic blood pressure cuffs (for this form you want to use the pulse from the lying or seated position). Some individuals have a pulse that skips beats. These individuals should understand that this is unacceptable, even though it is often seen by professionals as "normal." It's best to regard a skipping pulse as far from "ideal." This issue can be time sensitive enough to talk to a health coach.

Imbalance - Electrolyte Deficiency
- Low Blood Pressure (Resting Systolic BP < 112)
- Standing Diastolic BP < 73
- Pulse < 70
- Depression
- Vertigo
- Fatigue
- Insomnia
- Cravings

94

- Cramps (Hello? I assume most readers will add a check mark next to this one unless you just like to buy books about random topics, but this pertains to both menstrual cramps and muscle cramps, like charley horses. The majority of women reading this book will likely fall into this electrolyte deficiency category. Not all, but most. And most of you will be in this state due to a lack of digestion.)

Imbalance - Electrolyte Excess
- High Blood Pressure (Resting Systolic BP > 130)
- Standing Diastolic BP > 87
- Hypertension
- Cardiovascular Disease
- Poor Circulation

Circadian Rhythm (Cellular Permeability)

Imbalance - Anabolic
- Urine pH > 6.3
- Saliva pH < 6.6
- † Specific Gravity < 1.011
- Low Debris in Urine (This means that if you have your urine in a clear cup, you really won't see much floating around in there. Anabolic people are usually stuck in the rebuilding state, so they're not doing a lot of breaking down of old tissues or cells and the amount of debris found in the urine is much lower. You see the opposite under the catabolic state as a catabolic individual seems to always be peeing out junk the body is throwing away.)
- Hard Stool/Constipation
- High Body Temp
- Polyuria (Polyuria means frequent urination.)

- Difficult to Rise (Meaning the snooze button might be your best friend.)
- Anxiety
- Δ Adjusted Surface Tension > 69
- Δ Saliva mS < 4.5
- Δ Urine rH2 High (Surface tension, mS and rH2 are covered in Appendix A so I won't waste words explaining them here. If you can just flip to the back of the book instead of having me write it all out again, I can go have lunch now.)

Imbalance - Catabolic
- Urine pH < 6.1
- Saliva pH > 6.9
- † Specific Gravity > 1.020
- Soft/Loose Stool
- Oliguria (Infrequent urination, or frequent but in small amounts.)
- † Protein on Dipstick (This can be a strong catabolic marker because it's an indication that the body is breaking down tissues in the body. The protein that you're seeing here is protein from bodily tissues and usually not protein from a chicken sandwich.)
- Wake Easily
- Low Body Temp
- High Debris in Urine
- Insomnia
- Slow to Heal
- Migraines (A true migraine starts in the back of the head or the neck. The word "migraine" has come to describe any really bad headache, but not all headaches are truly migraines. If your headaches start at the front or top of your head, don't check this item.)
- Muscle Loss

- Δ Adjusted Surface Tension < 67
- Δ Saliva mS > 5.5
- Δ Urine rH2 Low

Energy Production

Imbalance - Tricarb Fast Oxidizer (Carb Burning)
- Breath Rate > 16bpm (The "bpm" stands for breaths per minute. Remember, each inhale counts as one. Don't count on both the inhale and the exhale.)
- Breath Hold < 50sec
- Low Blood Pressure (Resting Systolic BP < 112)
- Δ Glucose < 70 (I categorized this in the "need equipment" group, but you could do this test with a glucometer that can be picked up at any pharmacy.)
- Urine pH > 6.3
- Saliva pH < 6.6
- Fatigue
- Weight Issues
- Depression
- Irritable When Hungry

Imbalance - Beta Slow Oxidizer (Fat Burning)
- Breath Rate < 15bpm
- Breath Hold > 50sec
- High Blood Pressure (Resting Systolic BP > 133)
- Δ Glucose > 100
- Urine pH < 6.1
- Saliva pH > 6.9
- Fatigue
- Weight Issues
- Depression
- Type II Diabetes

Autonomic Nervous System

Imbalance - Parasympathetic

- Small Pupils
- Pulse Pressure < 37 (The pulse pressure is a measurement found by subtracting your Resting Diastolic BP number from your Resting Systolic BP number. This number is your pulse pressure. When you register on *The Coalition* and input your blood pressure numbers into the progress charts, the charts will automatically calculate your pulse pressure for you and display it on the graph as well.)
- Gag Reflex Increased (If you brush your teeth and your toothbrush goes a little further back, do you gag? When you go to the dentist, do you gag? Most women seem to know if they have a gag reflex or not.)
- Red Dermographic Line (This is the test I talked about in chapter four where you run the non-ink side of a pen across the inside of your arm and then wait 20-30 seconds to see if your skin turns red, white, or the mark just disappears. If the mark disappears, you don't need to add a check here. If it turns white, you'll place the check under "White Dermographic Line" in the Sympathetic section.)
- Low Body Temp (Below 98.6 degrees Fahrenheit. It should probably be at least a full point below or above before you would check this box or the high body temp box under sympathetic.)
- Warm Dry Hands
- Fingertips Warmer than Triceps (This is too hard to test on yourself since your triceps are the back of your upper arm, but you can have someone grab your fingertips and your triceps at the same time and tell you which is warmer. I recommend not having someone on the subway help you with this. Awkward.)

- Allergies
- Asthma

Imbalance - Sympathetic
- Large Pupils
- Pulse Pressure > 46
- Gag Reflex Decreased (You generally don't have a gag reflex.)
- White Dermographic Line
- High Body Temp
- Cold Hands
- Fingertips Colder than Triceps
- Dry Mouth
- Food Allergies

Acid/Alkaline Balance

Imbalance - Tending to Acidosis
- Breath Rate > 18bpm
- Breath Hold < 41sec
- Shortness of Breath

Imbalance - Tending to Alkalosis
- Breath Rate < 14bpm
- Breath Hold > 64sec
- Chronic Fatigue
- Sleep Apnea (Sleep apnea is where you wake up in the middle of the night because you weren't breathing. Oops.)

Digestive Issues
- Low Blood Pressure (Resting Systolic BP < 112)
- Standing Diastolic BP < 73

- Burping or Bloating (Many people don't really understand what bloating means. If you ask a woman, "Do your clothes fit tighter at night than when you put them on in the morning?" and she says, "Yes," she's bloating. As far as burping goes, I'm not talking about a huge belch. But if you have little burps after a meal, that is burping. Many people don't even notice that they burp until you ask them and they'll come back a day later and say, "Ya know, I really do burp.")
- Passing Gas
- Reflux/Heartburn
- Δ Total Ureas < 13
- Light Colored Stool (Either it is lighter than the color of corrugated cardboard, or your stool color will vary from light to dark depending on what you eat.)
- Constipation
- Urgent Diarrhea
- Nausea
- Δ rH2 > 20 or Δ rH2 < 17.5
- † Bilirubin on Dipstick

Okay, I Can Add Check Marks... Now What?

Once you've gone through the *Imbalance Guide* and added a check mark next to each piece of information that applies to you, you're ready to begin getting to know yourself. As you look over each imbalance box, the idea is just to see if one side has more check marks than the other side, and by how much. An entire box could have almost no check marks, or the check marks could be evenly distributed to both sides. Either of those options can be an indication of balance in that area. However, if you have more check marks on one side of an imbalance box than you do on the other side, that can be an indication of an area that could use some work. You're going to have to use your judgment here. Having one check mark on one side, and none on the other side, is hardly evidence of an imbalance. I really like to see at least a 30%

increase of the check marks on one side compared to the other side before I start to consider there to be any imbalance. Of course, I usually consider measurements to be more influential than symptoms in most cases.

Don't confirm an imbalance with just symptoms. If you have a few symptoms that are common for an imbalance, but none of your numbers point in that direction, I don't usually view that as enough to point me in any one direction. I really want to let the chemistry guide me and then use symptoms as tools of confirmation that the chemistry is an accurate picture. If an imbalance appears to be strong, go to the bottom of the *Imbalance Guide* and circle that imbalance. If it looks like you could be leaning that direction, but it's not so bad, you can just underline the imbalance to indicate that it needs work, but may not be your biggest trouble area. While evaluating your numbers, also look at how far out of range your numbers are. For example, if your systolic blood pressure is 89, that's a pretty long way from 112 so you can add more weight to that particular parameter. If your systolic blood pressure is 111, yes, that is still below range, but you may have just caught yourself at a low point and you'll want to test that number a couple more times over the next week or so.

When you test all your numbers, you're really looking at a range. You don't know if the day that you tested is an example of your best day or your worst day. That is why you will continue to check the easy tests a couple times a week so you can start to look for patterns in your numbers. If your systolic blood pressure is below 95 every time you test it, you know it's low. Just keep in mind that you're not using NASA equipment. It's just a blood pressure cuff you picked up at the pharmacy, right next to where they sell condoms that are ribbed for her enjoyment. It's probably not high-tech stuff or it wouldn't be sold right next to the contraceptive devices. You may often notice that you can check your blood pressure and see a systolic of 101 and then check it a few minutes later and see a systolic of 92. That's okay. Those are both low and you at least understand the range that you are in. It is the same with pH strips. You're using pH strips that are just indicating a measurement that you're interpreting through a color, you're not using a pH meter that's accurate to the hundredth.

What Is My Priority?

When it comes to deciphering which imbalance will be your priority, there are no absolute rules, only guidelines that will require you to use your judgment. Generally speaking, the imbalances above are listed in the order of their importance. In most cases, if you have an imbalance in your electrolytes box, that will take precedence over an imbalance in your cellular permeability box, energy production box or your autonomic nervous system box. However, if you have a fasting glucose of 275, you're not going to say I'll get to that later after I handle this Electrolyte Imbalance. Electrolytes may play a role in improving a high fasting glucose in the long term, but you're not going to want to ignore an issue as extreme as a fasting glucose approaching 300. I'm sure you can see how good sense and judgment could change your priorities when going over your *Imbalance Guide.*

You may also notice that the digestion box is located on the bottom of the page. But this is hardly your lowest priority. It's more of a baseline, since you will want to work on improving your digestion in the very beginning. Without your digestion working properly, working on imbalances is really futile, since the imbalances are likely expressing the way a starving system is compensating for its lack of nutrition. Not to mention, if digestion is not working properly, you may not be able to digest even a supplement correctly, in which case, how are you expected to make any progress with other imbalances?

Understanding Fluctuations In Your Numbers

Keep in mind that your chemistry is meant to change from one part of the day to the next. Your body is designed to be in a more catabolic state during the day and more of an anabolic state at night. If that oscillation from one state to the other is working correctly, you may see your pHs fluctuate from day to night. A "pH spread" is the difference between your urine pH and saliva pH. Having a large spread between a low urine pH and a high saliva pH can be an indication of a catabolic state. It's possible to see numbers in that range during the day, and then move to a more anabolic range at night (higher urine pH and lower saliva pH—where the spread between the two numbers would be smaller). If your numbers are stuck on one severe end of the spectrum, no matter what time of day it is, that may be a measurement worth paying special attention to while trying to figure out if you're dealing with an imbalance or not.

The goal is to find balance. If you have an Anabolic Imbalance, the goal is not to create a Catabolic Imbalance, you just want to move the body closer to balance. If you're using supplements and foods to help move you out of an imbalance, you just want to make sure you're monitoring your numbers and paying attention to what you're doing. You don't want to push so hard and so long that you create an imbalance of the opposite orientation. Once you start to see your numbers in the right place, I like to see people reduce the amount of supplements or reduce the specific foods that they are using to push themselves in that direction.

In chapter ten, I talk about how specific foods can help each imbalance. For now, just understand that you really need to be a participant in your own health and pay attention to your body. You don't, however, need to be a mad scientist and run numbers on yourself every fifteen minutes. That's not going to help and you're going to turn yourself into a nut-job. But some of the tests, like pHs and blood pressure, are very easy to look at. To run these tests once or twice a week is a reasonable and responsible thing to do. I mean, you're gonna pee every day anyway. Why not take a peek and see what is going on once in a while? Just keep your pH strips in your bathroom (but away from humidity) so you don't forget to use them. Then, simply keep track. That's why tools, like those *The Coalition* has put together, are so important for you to utilize.

Low Potassium Issues

Potassium in the body is a mineral that allows the cells to communicate back to the brain. It's what closes the control loop. The brain says, "Okay, let's do this" and then everybody down in the body communicates back to the brain, "Okay, this is what happened." Without enough potassium, the "this is what happened" doesn't make it back to the brain. Beyond the lack of coordination with your muscle/brain communication, low potassium issues can also cause a lack of coordination in the endocrine system.

When there is a low potassium issue, it's almost as if the body doesn't know what is going on since signals can't be properly transmitted. This can result in a variety of whacked out testing numbers. pHs can be all over the board and your test results might not make much sense at all.

Low potassium issues can be easier to detect with equipment and techniques used by a professional health coach. However, here are some signs you can look for that commonly coincide with low potassium issues:

- Food seen in your stool
- Burping or bloating
- Significant digestive issues
- Clumsiness
- Absent-minded or forgetful

If these issues sound familiar, you may want to be skeptical of your testing results. That doesn't mean that you should supplement potassium. The next step I would take would be to work on any digestive issues. Once you improve digestion, potassium can come into the system through your food. Good sources of extra potassium could be small green bananas, figs, a little black strap molasses, or orange juice. Just keep in mind that these are high carb foods, and high carb foods are not always the best idea when dealing with cramps.

Be Patient

I also want to explain that some things you do to move chemistry don't always show up immediately. That's not how the body works. You can't take a supplement or eat a specific food and expect your chemistry to be different an hour later, or even the next day. In that same line of thinking, you can't see a major change in your numbers and look at what you just did and think that was responsible. You can't say to yourself, "Well, I just watched an old episode of *Bewitched* and now my blood pressure is better." That's not how it works. You want the changes to your body to move slowly, just like agriculture does. Let me tell you a story to illustrate what I mean.

I was living in Florida and touring professionally as a comic. I was on a three-month trip all over the West Coast and still had a girlfriend on the East Coast. While I was working a week in Vegas, she flew out to see me. We were sitting at the buffet when we heard over the intercom, "Phone call for Mr. Knievel, Mr. Evel Knievel." We laughed at how someone must have gotten a hold of the intercom and was playing a joke. But that night, Evel Knievel came to my show and sat in the back of the room with my girlfriend. This part has nothing to do with my illustration, I just like to talk about Evel Knievel. The point of the story is that my girlfriend and I broke up on that trip. Not because she wanted me to be more dreamy, like Evel Knievel, but because with the long time away, we had just grown apart. The split was amicable but as I dropped her off at the airport, she couldn't stop crying. I was sad that we were splitting up, but I just wasn't emotional about it.

105

I returned to the airport the next morning for my flight back home, as my West Coast tour had ended and I missed all my rednecks in Florida. I got on the plane and sat in the middle seat between two very large men. Normally, when you sit down on a plane, you might share a few pleasantries or at least say, "Hi." For one reason or another, none of us said a word. I may have been silent just because I had already realized that I had about two feet available for me between both of these huge guys. About an hour into the flight, the cart started moving down the aisle to serve breakfast.

The stewardess, or sky frolicker, or whatever the current politically correct name is, set my breakfast on my foldout tray. I looked down to see two pieces of french toast, cut in half, with a sliced up pear in the middle. Pears were my girlfriend's favorite food. I looked down at the plate for about 30 seconds before tears started running down my face. By the time the air waitress had moved the cart down the aisle, I was sobbing like an eight-year-old girl that just smashed the cassette for her *Annie* soundtrack. It was full-on uncontrollable sobbing. Not cool. It lasted for more than a few minutes before the guy sitting to my right finally looked over and asked, "Are you okay?" I paused for a moment, collected myself, looked straight ahead and said to him with a trembling voice, "I just really like french toast." The guy to my left looked over to the guy to my right for a brief second, they both looked straight ahead just long enough to let what I said soak in, then we all went back to eating our breakfast and nobody said another word for the rest of the flight.

Do you see my point? I'm thinking that maybe you don't, but it's still a good story. My sobbing was not a result of the pears I just saw. There were layers upon layers of events, emotions and circumstances that led to me making a complete jackass out of myself on the plane that morning. That's how your body works. Just because you're trying to improve one imbalance doesn't mean that many layers of imbalances and chemistry are not being affected in many ways. With that in mind, try not to view a piece of information merely as cause and effect. It is often much more intricate than that and results will often take longer than you want them to take. Be patient. Your health is not an episode of *Miami Vice*. Everything will not be resolved in forty-five minutes.

Using The Coalition

In chapter four I introduced you to *The Coalition for Health Education*, which can be found at www.OurCoaltion.org. Since the annual membership fee to this private association is only $20 per year, I recommend joining to all those who plan on monitoring their own chemistry. The tools provided to members on *The Coalition* website are by far the best tracking and monitoring tools of their kind available to consumers. If you plan to use the guidelines presented in this book without monitoring your own chemistry, you're just a silly, silly person. Without watching what your numbers do, how are you going to know when to adjust the things you are implementing to balance your body? How are you going to know if you're making progress and how are you going to know when it's time to slow your efforts so you don't create an imbalance in the other direction? You have to monitor. You have to be a participant in your own health. A monitoring device is not something you own and ignore like the treadmill you hang your clothes on, it is something you actively use. The days of allowing someone to tell you, "Take these and come back to see me in two months," are over. You wouldn't be reading this book if you found that route worked for you. The sooner you come to the realization that you're going to have to put forth some effort, the sooner you'll improve your current circumstances and reap the rewards that come with responsible ownership of your own mechanism (by mechanism, I mean you).

Once you have an indication of what imbalances are giving you the most trouble, you can log in to your Coalition account and begin learning more about those imbalances and different ways to improve them. You can start to input your weekly self-test numbers into the progress charts to get a visual of how your numbers are moving and the progress you're making. There is even a graph for your "well-being" so you can monitor how the way you feel changes according to where your chemistry is. As you learn where your body seems to function optimally, you can start to get an idea of how to keep your chemistry in the place where you feel the best. Is that like cheating or what? I just love how sneaky that is, to look inside your own body and know exactly what is needed to feel your best. Who knew we would ever be able to do that?

The Coalition also provides you with a food journal system like no other. For each day, you can input what you're eating, how you're feeling, any symptoms that have come up or improved, etc. Then, when you enter self-test results in your progress charts, those results also show up in your food journal next to the appropriate time. Now, you can look at the foods you eat and see how those foods affect your chemistry and how you feel later that day. This can really help you pinpoint the foods and choices that are working best for you. No more throwing darts blindly at the menu of life. This can give you a clear-cut visual of the optimal diet for you... and you're in charge of the menu. I know I just said not to look at a food you just ate and then check your numbers and think that the food created those numbers. However, by watching what you eat over a few days at a time, and seeing how your numbers move, you can start to pick up patterns. That's what you're looking for—patterns.

The jewel of *The Coalition* is the pH balancing chart. This is some good stuff. Your urine pH has an optimal zone that changes according to your breath rate. If your breath rate is above sixteen, you will normally do well with a urine pH between 5.8 and 6.3 and a saliva pH between 6.5 and 7.0. If your breath rate is below 16, you will normally do well with a urine pH between 5.5 and 6.0 and a saliva pH between 6.5 and 7.0.

Optimal pHs According To Breath Rate

Breath Rate	Urine pH	Saliva pH
Above 16	5.8 – 6.3	6.5 – 7.0
Below 16	5.5 – 6.0	6.7 – 7.0

The pH balancing chart on *The Coalition* maps all that for you. Once you enter at least one urine pH entry and one saliva pH entry and one breath rate and breath hold entry, the system will create your pH balancing chart and display it within your personalized site. This chart will show you your optimal pH zones for both urine and saliva, and bring in your most recent pH entries from your progress charts so you can see if you're in your optimal zones or not. If you're out of your optimal zones, the chart lists foods and supplements that can help push those pHs in the right direction. It's an amazing tool and worth ten times the price of admission all by itself. Since I assisted *The Coalition* in creating this particular gadget, if it helps you improve your health as much as I believe it will, I think you should show your appreciation by sending me a new pair of flip-flops. I have a really hard time picking out flip-flops, but when they come to me as a gift I always seem to enjoy them.

Calling In A Professional

I've already gone on and on about how tricky this process can be. It's also tricky to rock a rhyme, to rock a rhyme that's right on time... it's tricky. But that's neither here nor there. The point I'm trying to impress upon you is to always remember that you are educating yourself about your body. Your body is a human body and it's just about the most amazing mechanism out there. (Other than a slinky. I just don't see how it does that thing down the stairs.) While you're working to better understand your body, keep in mind that *nobody* totally understands the human body. It's way too complicated. Remember that understanding these imbalances is complex enough, but when you start to realize that one imbalance on top of another can begin to change how the whole system is running, it can be a lot to sort through. I know there are people who will totally change their life by simply improving their digestion or a slight imbalance here or there, but a percentage of you will really need help from a professional to see major progress. The best part about plugging yourself into *The Coalition* and using their tracking tools is that you will be laying the groundwork in case you need to bring in a health coach to help you. When you contact *The Coalition* to find a professional in your area, and you begin to work with that person, *The Coalition* can then attach your account to that health coach. The coach will then be able to see all of your progress charts and how your chemistry has been moving with the efforts you have been putting in.

Presenting a new health coach with data that you have already been tracking can be a tremendous jump-start—not to mention the fact that you will understand your body enough now to have an intelligent conversation with the person who is guiding you in your education about your body. Unlike a doctor visit where you might not have a clue what he's talking about or why he's suggesting the things he is suggesting, if you've read this book and you've been monitoring your chemistry on *The Coalition*, you will be miles ahead of the game. It will be so much easier for you to be a participant in your own health.

CHAPTER SIX

Imbalances

Imbalances And Your Symptoms

As a society, we are deeply entrenched in the mindset of looking at our symptoms and trying to find "remedies" to address those symptoms. The difficult task I will bestow upon you while reading this book is to take that train of thought and smash it into a wall. In order to truly find balanced health, you need to look *beyond* the symptom to what is causing the symptom.

Most symptoms are the result of one or more imbalance. Some symptoms will commonly show up in an individual who is suffering from a specific imbalance or a combination of imbalances. With that understanding, we can use symptoms as information to help us get a better picture of which imbalances may be affecting our body the most. But we should look at those symptoms only as a piece of data and not as the deciding factor. One symptom, say insomnia, can be the result of three or four different imbalances.

If you were to try to treat your symptom of insomnia, you could be throwing darts for months and missing every time. However, if you look at an imbalance that you are experiencing, and that imbalance is one that commonly creates insomnia, now you've got something. Now, you can just focus on correcting that imbalance and the symptom that goes along with it will often improve as well. As a bonus, you may even see other problems that you are not as distressed about begin to improve too.

With this insight, it can be beneficial for you to take into account which symptoms may be causing you the most trouble, just be sure to use that information only as a clue instead of allowing it to steer your ship. If you steer your ship with your symptoms, you're going to have a pissed off ship. Gaining knowledge of the imbalances below will be your first step toward understanding how the human body operates and how to operate your human body.

Each imbalance may show itself in the form of a number of different symptoms or conditions. The outcome may be different depending on the individual, but many of the imbalances I describe have symptoms that will commonly show up for people with these imbalances. Therefore, under each imbalance I list some of the symptoms that can show up when that imbalance is present. But if you read about the symptoms that can show up with one imbalance, and you jump to the conclusion that you have that imbalance before you even test yourself, I'm going to make this book self-destruct and you won't get to read it anymore. Don't do that. Don't put yourself in a category because of symptoms. The only way to know where you are is to look at your numbers, like I taught you in chapter four.

Now that I've given you a time out, you can continue reading, but only with the awareness that the symptoms listed under each imbalance are not a confirmation of that imbalance. I'm just listing issues that can commonly show up when each imbalance is present. I still don't know which sibling left my Scooby-Do lunchbox in the sun until it melted. This has created some trust issues and I won't be able to count on you to remember this "symptoms rule." Please forgive me if I remind you again in this section. However, I don't want to treat you like a six-year-old either so I'm not going to bring it up after each topic. I think I've been annoying about this point enough for now and we can all move on with our lives.

Electrolyte State

The electrolyte state is defined by blood pressure (though a professional health coach may have equipment that can look at other variables in this equation, like conductivity of urine and saliva). When blood pressure is low, this is often a reflection of low mineral content in the bloodstream. When the mineral levels decrease, it is a reflection of a decrease in your salts or the vascular system being too open (dilated). Our mineral content not only comes from actual salt, but from our food too. If your digestion is not working properly, you can't assimilate the minerals from the food you're eating and the mineral content in the system can decrease. (I go over this in more detail when I talk about digestion in chapter seven.) There are a few other possible contributing factors that can result in low blood pressure and I will get back to this soon. In most cases, however, digestion is the most prevalent contributing factor to low blood pressure. When we see low blood pressure, for example, anything lower than a systolic reading (the top number) of 112 and a diastolic reading (the bottom number) lower than 73, we consider that there is likely an Electrolyte Deficiency Imbalance present.

Imbalance - Electrolyte Deficiency

Very few doctors will ever complain about your blood pressure being low. Since there is no drug for low blood pressure, the ramifications are not in their training. We all know that high blood pressure can cause heart attacks and strokes (blowouts). When they say your blood pressure is great even though it's too low, they're saying that you'll never have a blowout. But is it fun to run around on flat tires all day? An optimal blood pressure reading is said to be 120 over 80. So, if 140 over 90 is considered high blood pressure in the medical world, wouldn't having those numbers off by the same amount in the other direction be regarded as low blood pressure? Shouldn't a reading of 100 over 70 be considered low?

The minerals, or salts, in the system represent the conductivity, or ability for electricity to flow through the system. When the mineral content is low, there's no spark and energy can be low. Without this energy, the brain can't function at its full potential, a result created by the lack of minerals required for signals to travel through. Many people with depression, and even other manifestations of "mental illness," are often just cases where there is not enough mineral in the system. Low mineral levels often mean there's not enough spark to give the brain what it needs to function correctly, or there is not enough mineral to control blood pH sufficiently. Of course, blood sugar is a big player in this regard also, but I get into that in a bit.

We sort of have this mindset that, if what we're eating is providing us with enough energy to stand up and walk to our car, we have all the resources we need. But every task that our bodies handle needs resources to complete it. Vitamins, minerals, amino acids—they're all important. The mineral in the system is very important because, without it, there is no way for signals to travel from the body to the brain. It's like electricity in water. If you put an electrical current in water, you get shocked and it's really not that fun. You get shocked because that water contains minerals and that current can travel through them. But if you put a current in distilled water, with no mineral in it, the current doesn't travel. It's the same way with your brain. If signals can't travel, the brain doesn't work optimally and we feel depressed, tired or lethargic, or in the worst cases, maybe we think that we're a fire truck. Almost all of the clients with depression issues that have come to me, or to any of my colleagues, have shown a low blood pressure reading (unless they are taking an anti-depressant that is raising their blood pressure artificially). There are exceptions to every rule. I mean just the other day I saw a guy with a mullet that actually looked good, so there can be a first time for everything.

But generally speaking, the majority of clients I see with depression symptoms have low blood pressure.

The brain needs fuel just like anything else. If your toaster isn't working, what's the first thing you check? You look to see if it's plugged in. You don't send your toaster to therapy or soak it in medication; you just look to see if it's getting the juice it needs to function properly. I'm not saying that therapy can't be beneficial for some people, I'm just saying that, when it comes to mechanical objects, we have the sense to look at a malfunction and try to figure out what is causing that object to function inadequately. However, when it comes to people, we don't check to see if the person has the resources for their "machine" to perform optimally. We just assume they must have daddy abandonment issues, or felt inadequate as a child because their brother was always the first one to find the prize in the bottom of the cereal box. Yes, it can be very upsetting to think back on the terror of your brother having fun with all the press-on tattoos while you had none, but if your brain had the resources to function at its full potential, it would be easier to look past that and move on with your life, now that you're 36.

Don't feel like I'm downplaying depression issues just because I'm talking like a jackass. I've experienced these issues first-hand and they can be very troubling, confusing, and a huge pile of not-at-all-fun. They were especially confusing for me because I had always been a very positive person; then all of a sudden, I just wanted to ball up on the floor and cry at old episodes of *The Brady Bunch*. Once I understood how these issues can come out of nowhere, what imbalances most often create them and how to improve those imbalances, I was right back to my old self and could once again laugh at the fact that it *WAS* Mom's favorite vase and she *DID* always say don't play ball in the house. (Non-Brady fans will have no idea what I'm talking about here and may think I'm a little drunk right now.) You can learn more about why this happens and how to improve these issues in my upcoming book, *Kick Depression in the Nuts*. But for now, we just want to lay down

115

a foundation that can help you understand how the body needs nourishment to do all the things it does. The body can't just show up to work every day and make it all magically happen. Resources are needed to keep your "machine" running properly.

Cravings

I promised I would at least touch on the topic of cravings. This can be a very complicated issue, with many different contributing factors, and I will go over all of them when I release my book, *Kick Cravings in the Nuts*. I'm going to talk about just one of the possible causes here, but it happens to be the most common and dominating cause for cravings when it comes to sugar or chocolate. Just by following the guidelines in this book to improve your cramps, most of you will never need to read *Kick Cravings in the Nuts* because you will have already improved the issue by accident while you were doing the work to improve your cramps. If that's not a free bonus, I don't know what is.

Cravings can be a touchy subject for some people and a tough issue they have dealt with for years, or even decades. Yes, there can be emotional baggage attached to cravings that go all the way back to your first Easy-Bake Oven, or even earlier. But if you have emotional issues and are in need of finding a way past them, understanding what I'm about to explain to you can take the difficulty level of moving past them from a ten, all the way down to a one... if you're willing to do the work to correct this one circumstance. Here is how it works. If a person's salts (mineral content) are low, that person can have seizures. If a person's sugars are low, that person can have seizures. If salts and sugars are low at the same time, that person has an even greater chance of having a seizure. If your blood pressure is usually low, and you have other issues that can push your blood sugar very low too, that's the perfect recipe for some crazy, crazy cravings—the type of cravings where you might literally steal candy from a baby. (I'm sure you rationalized it by saying that the baby was very whiny and did not deserve the candy.)

116

When I get to the Anabolic/Catabolic Imbalances section, I explain the imbalance that can cause blood sugars to go too low. When a person's minerals and sugars go too low at the same time, this is the most common cause for cravings. This is usually why people crave salty foods, sweet and sugary foods, or carbs like bread or crackers (that can be converted to sugars). The body isn't so dumb. If salts are low, you can buffer them by raising your sugars and you'll be fine. The reverse is also true. If sugars are low, you can buffer them by raising your salts. The cravings are just your body's way of helping you to raise either your salts or your sugars in order to keep you from pushing toward seizures.

Where most people think that something is wrong with them, or they just have no willpower, the truth is you can't compete with a body that knows how to get what it needs to continue functioning properly. Does that mean that these sugars or carbs are good for you? No; but don't you think your body would be more concerned with not having seizures than it would be with gaining weight or augmenting your cramps? Doesn't it make sense that if the body recognized a "looming seizure" that was basically going to shut down the whole system, it would take some steps to keep that from happening?

To get rid of cravings, people with low salts can raise their mineral content by:

1. Using unrefined salt (like sea salt).
2. Using specific supplements.
3. Correcting any digestion problems that are keeping the body from properly breaking down food, so the mineral content can be assimilated by the body. If you're not digesting correctly, you're not getting the minerals out of your food.

I go over all those steps in detail after you are able to look at your specific body chemistry and figure out which of those steps, or what combination of those steps, are appropriate for you.

117

Just don't get ahead of me. I'm not saying that if you're craving sugar you're about to have a seizure. It just means the body is very defensive when it comes to having seizures, and it plans way ahead of time by sending out the signal for more things that can thicken the bloodstream and raise the minerals or the sugars. Your body doesn't know that you have cereal in the cupboard thirty feet away. It still operates under the assumption that you need to go out and hunt down a zebra or track down berries somewhere. Believe it or not, the body was not designed with "Special K" in mind.

The body may be feeling a little panicked about the low resources. The body may be sending the signal that you interpret as, "Hey... you... go to the store and get some double fudge ice cream and a box of those Nilla Wafers." This urge doesn't mean that a seizure is about to kick in. Even if you didn't eat anything else for another ten to twenty hours or more, you likely could still avoid a seizure. Tricking your brain into thinking that ordering a pizza and a box of doughnuts is a good idea is not the only backup maneuver your body has when resources are low. When your body is not getting the nutrients it needs, it will often just steal those nutrients from your own tissues or bones. The body will literally mine itself for what it needs in order to survive. Of course, after twenty years of mining for what it needs, this backup plan can become less and less successful for the body as resources become more depleted. The optimal idea is to simply give your body what it needs in the first place.

I've seen this information about why people experience cravings totally transform lives. I've had clients who were going to therapy for over a decade, just for their cravings. When they learned how to raise the mineral content in their body and give their body what it really needs, those cravings just stopped... like I was magic or maybe even a leprechaun of some sort. (Why do you have to laugh at that like it was a short joke? You don't know how short I am. Maybe I'm very, very tall. Maybe I was the tallest guy in my school and nobody picked on me or stole my Chewbacca action figure... Okay, I don't want to talk about that anymore.)

Possible symptoms that can show up with an Electrolyte Deficiency Imbalance:
- chronic fatigue
- low blood pressure
- menstrual cramps
- poor circulation
- decreased libido
- depression or anxiety
- vertigo or dizziness when standing
- cravings
- insomnia

Imbalance - Electrolyte Excess

If an Electrolyte Deficiency Imbalance normally indicates a lack of electrolytes, the opposite would be a state where too many electrolytes are present. This is called an Electrolyte Excess Imbalance. In the world of natural health, where the terrain of the body gives so many insights into how the body is functioning, if an imbalance can exist in one direction, there must be an opposite to that imbalance. Otherwise, there would be no middle ground, no place where the body could be considered "balanced." Seems reasonable, right? By the time you finish this book, you will likely realize how ridiculous it is that the medical world puts so much attention on high blood pressure, but totally ignores an equally severe imbalance in the other direction.

In general, high blood pressure can be an expression of insufficient, or lousy, kidney function. This means that, when excessive electrolytes become concentrated in the bodily fluids, it's usually a result of insufficient hydration (not drinking enough clean water) or impaired excretion of mineral salts through the kidneys. High blood pressure can also result from a constricted vascular system. In any case, electrolyte stress can lead to hypertension (high blood pressure) and other circulatory and cardiovascular problems. A vascular system that is constricted often points to an autonomic nervous system issue or a buildup on the arterial walls. (I talk more about the autonomic nervous system when I talk about Sympathetic and Parasympathetic Imbalances.)

Stiffening arterial walls can lift pulse pressure, which is the difference between the systolic and diastolic blood pressure numbers. When the pulse pressure becomes greater and greater as the arterial walls become stiffer and stiffer, the heart becomes weaker and weaker. If you are a person with high blood pressure who is trying to bring it down naturally, watching the pulse pressure correct itself helps to validate that you are doing the right thing. Remember, *The Coalition for Health Education* has a tool that calculates your pulse pressure for you so you can just monitor the changes without worrying about the math or really understanding what pulse pressure is.

You can read more about high blood pressure when I release, *Kick High Blood Pressure in the Nuts*. Since most of the issues that can contribute to menstrual cramps lean more toward an Electrolyte Deficiency Imbalance than toward an Electrolyte Excess Imbalance, in this book, I talk more about the former.

Possible symptoms that can show up with an Electrolyte Excess Imbalance:
- high blood pressure
- hardening of the arteries
- heart attack
- stroke
- poor circulation
- inability to properly transport oxygen, nutrients, waste products, antibodies and more, throughout your system

Cellular Permeability

At the cellular level, the body is always in an anabolic or catabolic state, or in the process of switching back and forth between the two. During the day, our cell membranes are intended to open up (much like a flower) so nutrients can get in and out more easily. This "more open" state is called a catabolic state. At night, our cell membranes are intended to become more closed (again, like a flower) so nutrients cannot get in and out as easily. This "more closed" state is called an anabolic state. The anabolic and catabolic states, at the cellular level, are as obvious a fact as day and night on Earth or tides in the ocean. Both states are appropriate, and even necessary, for a body to function optimally. Due to many possible factors, some people can get stuck in one state and their body will not switch back and forth like it is intended to.

Our cells are made up of different types of fats: fatty acids and sterols. If there are too many sterols in the cell membrane, and not enough fatty acids, the body can be predisposed to become stuck in an anabolic state (as previously described). With too many fatty acids and not enough sterols, we could be predisposed to get stuck in a catabolic state (the opposite of an anabolic state). To make the body operate correctly, we need to oscillate back and forth from the anabolic state at night, while we sleep, and a catabolic state during the day, while we're active. Without this natural oscillation, many problems can occur. When the body shifts from anabolic to catabolic, that's when the endorphins in the brain are released, which can help people from becoming depressed. I will talk about this more in one of my next books, *Kick Depression in the Nuts*. Though there are many other factors that more commonly contribute to depression, you can see that this natural oscillation between the anabolic and catabolic states can be important. Let's go over each of these imbalances individually for a minute. You cool with that?

Imbalance - Anabolic

First of all, there are many benefits that take place while a body is in an anabolic state. This is the state where the body engages in most of its repairing or rebuilding processes. You've probably heard the word anabolic in reference to steroids. Weightlifters take anabolic steroids in order to be in the tissue building, anabolic state when they are not playing fair with muscle building. If a guy begins to add some muscle and thinks, "This is nice, but I'd really like to be so big that my neck completely disappears and I can no longer hold my arms down at my sides. I want my arms to always look like they are sticking straight out like Ralphie's little brother, Randy, from *A Christmas Story* when he was wearing his winter parka. That's what I want to look like." By using these anabolic steroids, this guy can keep his body in an anabolic, muscle building state most of the time. It's true that he may not be thinking about the fact that these steroids are going to make everything on his body bigger except the one thing he truly wants to be bigger. If you think about it, isn't making everything else bigger just going to make that "one thing" seem smaller. C'mon guys, think it through before you make yourself look like an alien action figure.

I'm not trying to get as many Hulk-looking guys as possible to want to crush me. What I am trying to do is point out that, while an anabolic state can have its benefits, any state can cause problems when pushed to an extreme—even problems beyond becoming so huge that you look more like a video game character than a human. Although it is very appropriate for the cells to be in an anabolic state at night, some individuals will stay in a more anabolic state most of the time. These individuals are said to be experiencing an Anabolic Imbalance.

If you're stuck in an anabolic state most of the time, it can be very hard to get up in the morning because your body, at the cellular level, is actually still in sleep mode. In the same way that many people who suffer from insomnia are stuck in a catabolic state where their body is always awake, anabolic people can have a hard time getting their bodies in motion in the morning. The snooze button can be their best friend. Be sure to understand, however, that everyone who experiences insomnia is not necessarily stuck in a catabolic state. You will soon be able to read more about this topic in *Kick Insomnia in the Nuts*. Just don't think that, if you suffer from insomnia, you must not have an Anabolic Imbalance because a Catabolic Imbalance is only one possible cause for insomnia. There are insomnia cases that exist quite well in an anabolic state too. Also, don't think that if you pop right out of bed in the morning that you can't have an Anabolic Imbalance. Throughout this book, be sure to remember that imbalances can show their heads in different ways for different people. There are no "rules" to follow, only guidelines to help you along.

This Anabolic Imbalance can also cause constipation by sending too much of the body's water to the kidneys and not enough to the bowels, making the stool harder and more difficult to move. An Anabolic Imbalance can also cause individuals to pee high volumes of urine frequently throughout the day. They will often have to get up in the middle of the night to tinkle.

Possible symptoms that can show up with an Anabolic Imbalance:
- constipation or hard stool
- tachycardia (rapid heart rate)
- anxiety / panic attacks
- frequent urination
- difficulty waking in the morning
- viral problems

Since an overly anabolic state can be described as a lack of fatty acids at the cellular level, increasing your fatty acid intake can be one method to help improve this imbalance. However, I find that most individuals with this imbalance really need to use more nutrients like specific vitamins, minerals and amino acids, more than fatty acids, in order to see lasting improvement. Increasing your fatty acid intake may be a place to start when attempting to improve an Anabolic Imbalance, but wait until I talk about supplements in chapters eleven through thirteen before you go out and buy all kinds of fatty acid supplements. They are not all created equal and taking rancid fatty acid supplements can be more harmful than good. Yes, mainstream media loves to cram the benefits of fatty acids down our throats; but not only are fatty acids not beneficial for some imbalances, rancid fatty acids are not beneficial for anyone. (Here comes one of those reminders I warned you about.)

Beyond buying the right supplements, also be sure not to just assume you have an imbalance because you're experiencing some (or even all) of the symptoms that commonly show up with that imbalance. Without looking at your specific chemistry, and understanding how your body is operating, you're really just throwing darts when you try to treat symptoms that way. There are thousands of books out there on how to treat symptoms and you can get through them a lot faster because you'll be avoiding all the "jackass-laden" analogies that I like to make people read in my books for my own enjoyment. With that in mind, if you want to treat symptoms, you should read one of those books. If you want to get results, be patient, keep reading, and wait until you understand where your body really is before you run out to the health food store and buy something new every three or four pages, just because it *sounds* like it might help you.

Imbalance - Catabolic

When it comes to cellular permeability, the catabolic state is the opposite of the anabolic state. It's the other side of the coin. The catabolic state is where the body kind of "breaks down and cleans house," so to speak. In a catabolic state, the body is primed to use oxygen to create energy, so it is appropriate to be in a catabolic state during your waking hours to keep you going all day. This, along with what I just explained about the anabolic state, helps to show how both the anabolic and catabolic states are appropriate during the appropriate times. However, in the same way that we talked about people who lean too anabolic, some individuals will stay in a more catabolic state most of the time. These individuals are said to be experiencing a Catabolic Imbalance.

If someone is stuck in a catabolic state, the cell walls are too permeable and this individual will often burn up muscle and protein and even membrane fats. Breaking down tissues and muscle so they can be rebuilt is a beneficial aspect of the catabolic state, but when a person is in that state too often, for too long, that "cleaning house" process can turn into a body that is flat out falling apart. If you bulldoze your garage to add on a new wing to your house, your house could increase its value. But if you knock down your garage just because you're addicted to knocking things down, your neighbors won't like you, just like you won't like your body if you're unable to move back into that "rebuilding" state. The more muscle we lose, the lower our metabolism, and we may burn less fat.

Insomnia is very common in catabolic people because their cell membranes are more permeable, which is a characteristic of the daytime state. These people can't sleep because their bodies are still awake and operating at full speed. Most sleeping aids will knock you out in the head so you can sleep, but your body will still be wide awake all night. As a result, you might either wake up exhausted or you become tired again a few hours after waking. I guess it depends on your candle, and how short it has become by burning both ends at once. The point is, I'd like to teach you how to fix the problem instead of just selling you more candles.

Possible symptoms that can show up with a Catabolic Imbalance:
- insomnia
- migraines
- chronic diarrhea or loose stool
- hair falling out
- muscle loss

- chronic pain
- loss of connective tissue or difficulty in healing
- aging quickly
- joint and muscle pain; arthritis (especially rheumatoid)
- oliguria (insufficient urination, perhaps often but in small amounts)
- low body temperature
- bacterial problems

Since an overly catabolic state is sometimes described as a lack of sterols at the cellular level, increasing your intake of sterols and saturated fatty acids, such as real butter or coconut oil, can be one method to help improve this imbalance. However, I find that most individuals with this imbalance also need to use more nutrients like specific vitamins, minerals and amino acids in order to see lasting improvement. That being said, increasing your sterol intake while optimizing digestion can be a great place to start.

Energy Production

The next two imbalances I cover are Beta Oxidizer Imbalance and Tricarb Oxidizer Imbalance. These deal with energy production and how the body uses food for fuel. Before I explain energy production, understand that I will be leaving out complicated methods the body can use to create energy. They are not important for this explanation and I would like to finish up and leave before my cleaning lady gets here. She dresses inappropriately for a cleaning lady and it freaks me out.

To create energy, simply speaking, our bodies burn either fat or glucose. Your body is designed to burn both types of fuel for different purposes. Despite that, changes can occur in our bodies, or in our lives, that will train our bodies to prefer one fuel over the other. The body may stop burning the other type of fuel almost entirely. This is another reason why there is no such thing as the diet that is right for everyone. It doesn't exist. You have a better chance of finding an insightful Vin Diesel movie than you have of finding a diet that will be appropriate for every person. Some people burn fats much better than glucose and some people are the opposite. This really puts all these arguments into perspective about "low-carb," "low-fat," "high-protein," "the ice cream sandwich diet," "I only eat things that start with the letter F..." I could go on for days. They're still all going to be wrong. In order to find the right "diet," you really need to look at the person, because each person processes foods differently.

Imbalance - Tricarb Oxidizer

Tricarbs are people who are predisposed to burn off all their glucose and do not seem to burn fat very well. Now, it's not that they won't burn fat, but they will always prefer to burn off all their glucose first. This is commonly referred to as hypoglycemic. Just keep in mind that the hypoglycemic can also be a step away from becoming diabetic. "But if he's hypoglycemic, how can he be a step away from becoming diabetic?" It's because many hypoglycemics have way too much insulin in the system and their system responds as though there are five furnaces in the house. Every time the house gets cold, instead of one furnace coming on and slowly warming up the house and then turning off, FIVE furnaces turn on and the house is hot enough to make you cuss by the time the furnaces shut down.

A tricarb's insulin can work in this same manner. These individuals have become insulin resistant, but they have not been insulin resistant long enough that the cells have stopped responding to the insulin altogether. They're at that stage where the cells are still responsive enough to the insulin that, when the pancreas produces up to five times the amount of insulin it normally would, it reaches a critical level and all the sugar goes into the cells at one time. These people can get very severe headaches in the front of their heads. They may also complain that their head feels full or they'll get fuzzy brained; this is due to

127

the blood sugar dropping far too rapidly. Using a blood sugar glucometer can quantify that the blood glucose has gone too low. This low blood sugar can make these folks extremely miserable, and being around them when blood sugar levels drop can be equally miserable. If you live with, or if you are this person, you know exactly what I'm talking about.

Possible symptoms that can show up with a Tricarb Oxidizer Imbalance:
- lack of energy; physical and mental fatigue
- high or low blood sugar
- shortness of breath
- high cholesterol
- overweight or underweight
- irritable when hungry

Imbalance - Beta Oxidizer

If you find that you show indications of having a Beta Oxidizer Imbalance, you most likely are burning much more fat than glucose. If you also have high cholesterol, high triglycerides and a high fasting glucose, any of these markers can be another indication that you are not processing glucose effectively.

Many individuals who are overweight and have this imbalance will ask, "How is it that I'm burning mostly fat but I'm still so fat?" This is because their bodies are turning almost every carb and sugar that they eat into fat. In order to process sugar or glucose, the body is having to take all sugar or glucose coming into a person and turn it into fat before it is able to be "burned" for energy.

Possible symptoms that can show up with a Beta Oxidizer Imbalance:
- lack of energy; physical and mental fatigue
- Type II Diabetes

- metabolic syndrome (or insulin resistance)
- high blood pressure or cardiovascular disease
- weight gain
- gallbladder trouble

You may have noticed Type II Diabetes on the list above. This doesn't mean that if you have a Beta Oxidizer Imbalance that you're diabetic. It just means that in this Beta Oxidizer state, the body prefers to burn fat and can often move into a predicament where it will burn very little glucose, if any. In these cases, glucose can accumulate in the bloodstream and, abracadabra, you're diabetic. Remember, I am only describing an imbalance in this section and not a disease. However, a neglected imbalance certainly can manifest itself eventually as a disease, just like neglecting to change the oil in your engine can manifest itself as a blown up engine.

By improving this imbalance and allowing the body to once again process both types of fuel, a person could increase energy and lose some weight, since such a large percentage of glucose would no longer need to be stored as fat.

Autonomic Nervous System

Sympathetic Dominance refers to the autonomic nervous system (ANS). The ANS is a mechanism in the body that happens without having to consciously think about it. You don't have to think about whether your heart is beating, it just does. The other side of the nervous system is the Parasympathetic Dominance, or the part of the nervous system that you can control.

The sympathetic side is the speed side—the fight or flight response. The parasympathetic side is the slow side—the rest and digest state. These two systems are hard-wired, in a sense, to the heart, the entire digestive system, and all the lower level glands, organs and systems.

Imbalance - Parasympathetic

A Parasympathetic Imbalance is often where I find individuals who suffer from allergies or asthma. This can be a tricky imbalance because if an individual has a strong ANS imbalance, especially on the parasympathetic side, that person can often see a response that is opposite of what is expected when working to balance the body. For example, if a specific food or supplement tends to push one measurement, like urine pH, down for most people, that same food or supplement could actually push up that measurement for a parasympathetic person. I've never heard a good explanation as to why this can occur for some, but this anomaly is seen frequently enough in parasympathetics that you need to know this anomaly exists. That is why learning to monitor your body is so important. Monitoring your body will also alert you when the time has come to get the help of a professional who understands the wide variety of nuances that can occur when looking at layer upon layer of imbalances in the body.

Possible symptoms that can show up with a Parasympathetic Imbalance:
- allergies
- asthma
- small pupil size
- frequent urination
- increased saliva
- muscle cramps at night
- eyes or nose watery
- eyelids swollen
- gag easily
- poor circulation

Imbalance - Sympathetic

The ANS is reactive. As a stress situation presents itself, the system turns on, does its job, and in doing so possibly reaches its outer bounds of homeostasis (perfect balanced health). Thanks to this selfish act of the ANS, other systems in the body can be deprived and suffer. Not unlike the transmission in your car, systems in the body can "lock up" and refuse to shift out of low gear, thus causing a myriad of symptoms such as unpredictable and/or uncalled-for behavior. The stress situations that are instigating the reaction of the ANS could be emotional, nutritional, or mineral in origin. If individuals are stuck in a sympathetic state, they can feel stressed and on edge, and even have trouble sleeping since they are stuck in fight or flight mode.

Possible symptoms that can show up with a Sympathetic Imbalance:
- large pupil size
- low levels of urination
- increased temperature
- sweaty hands
- dry mouth/eyes/nose
- get chills often
- cold extremities (like hands or feet)
- unable to relax
- irritated by strong light

pH Balance

Everybody just calm down. This can be a very hot topic in the world of natural health. If this book is your first taste of natural health, this section may open your eyes to some incredible things. Kind of like the series *LOST*, but this will actually make sense. However, if you have already read, or have been introduced to, information about the pH of the body, I may need to spend some time fixing the damage that some other numskulls have created.

In the natural world, when people talk about pH, they frequently talk about how we all need to "alkalize." "Alkalize, alkalize, alkalize." "Alkalize or die a slow, miserable death," they tell us. These pH "gurus" explain how we are all too "acid" and it's killing us one by one. Of course, when someone follows these approaches and tries to alkalize themselves, and they completely fall apart, the guru tells them, "That's okay, you're going through a 'healing crisis'. Just stick to it and you'll be fine." No, what we're going through is a guru crisis. There currently appears to be a crisis where a few gurus need to be punched in the neck so maybe they will stop ruining the well-being of half of their readership.

These readers who started to fall apart after "alkalizing" themselves were likely falling apart because they were pushing an imbalance that already existed even further over the edge. Remember how I talked about the fact that an imbalance can't exist unless there is an equal imbalance in the other direction? If someone told you one pair of glasses will fix everyone's vision, you would question his intelligence or just poke him in the eye. We all know that reading glasses can help farsighted people while nearsighted individuals need the very opposite type of lens. Any author who tells the reader that EVERYONE should do ANYTHING is trying to sell something. It's also possible that said author is just dumb, understands that they're dumb, and wants somebody to tell them that they're smart. If that's the case, here you go... "You're so smart, Buddy." Now, leave those poor people alone and quit making them worse.

The haphazard confusion starts here; some individuals truly are too "acidic." I talk about what this means in just a moment. For now, I'm going to continue using the same ignorant terminology that most of the pH gurus use. When individuals have an Acid Imbalance, and they truly can benefit from "alkalizing" themselves, these individuals can follow the instructions laid out by a pH guru and they may see tremendous improvement to their health, or at least their well-being. In some cases, these results could even be considered miraculous. Still, let's just calm down for a minute. If we know that every imbalance (like an Acid Imbalance) will have an opposite imbalance in the other direction, what are these pH gurus doing to the people who have an Alkaline Imbalance (the opposite of an Acid Imbalance)? They're making these individuals miserable and calling it a "healing crises," that's what they're doing.

To go right along with all of the pH and alkalizing books and experts out there, we also find shelves upon shelves of "alkalizing" products in every health food store. You can't throw a stick down the aisle of a health food store without hitting a product that boasts its ability to improve your health through alkalizing. (By the way, if you do this, the employees will come right up to you and ask you not to throw sticks in their store anymore... like I'm the one doing something wrong here.) It is also likely that these products will increase in popularity since many people will reap benefits from their use. Many people with an acidity issue, that is. To understand the tragedy in this, let's go over the Acid and Alkaline Imbalances.

The most important thing to understand is that, when I discuss an Acid or Alkaline Imbalance in this series of books, I am talking about blood pH. Measuring urine pH and saliva pH in a context of breath rate and breath hold can be incredibly insightful and useful, but urine pH or saliva pH are not always an indication of the pH of the blood, as many pH gurus will have you believe. It's a nice story, it just happens to be a fictional one. I already showed you how to measure urine pH and saliva pH, and later in the book I talk even more about what these measurements can indicate when it comes to how your body is operating. For now, I'm just going to dig into blood pH since this is the crucial parameter when looking at an Acid or Alkaline Imbalance.

Imbalance - Tending to Alkalosis

The bloodstream has a very narrow pH value that it must stay within in order for our bodies to function properly. If the blood moves too far acid or too far alkaline, we can literally die. The body doesn't want this to happen, so it does whatever it can to keep the bloodstream at a balanced pH level. Alkalosis is an imbalance where the bloodstream is too alkaline. When the blood leans alkaline, oxygen can't leave the bloodstream and go to the tissue level where it needs to be to help your body create the energy required to run properly. In science, this is known as the Bohr Effect.

If a doctor checked your oxygen levels, he would put a device called a pulse oximeter on you and he might tell you that your oxygen is great... you have plenty. But, because the bloodstream is too alkaline, the oxygen cannot be released from the bloodstream and go into the tissues where it can be used. The result: You can feel wiped out. The oxygen is there, it just can't get to the right location in order to be properly utilized. In an effort to correct this, when the bloodstream is too alkaline, the body will slow the rate at which you breathe. Carbon dioxide (CO_2) is acid inducing to the bloodstream so the body tries to reduce the amount that you breathe in order to hold on to more CO_2, allowing it to acidify the bloodstream. Pretty neat trick Mother Nature came up with, don't you think? By using the CO_2 to acidify a bloodstream that is too alkaline, some oxygen can be released from the bloodstream and make it to the tissue level.

Possible symptoms that can show up with an Alkaline Imbalance:
- chronic fatigue
- sleep apnea
- joint and muscle pain; arthritis
- allergies; asthma
- muscle cramps
- fluid retention

In regard to sleep apnea, many cases are caused by structural issues (such as a flap that doesn't seem to be flapping correctly), but almost as many are caused by a bloodstream that is too alkaline. The breath rate drops so low due to an overly alkaline bloodstream that eventually the body says, "I'm gonna acidify this bloodstream and get some oxygen down to the tissues where it needs to be even if it kills this guy," and this would show itself as sleep apnea symptoms.

By looking at all the trouble an overly alkaline bloodstream can cause, do you see how important it is to look at people as individuals and measure where they are before you start blabbing about how everyone needs to alkalize? Just because something brings about an amazing result for one person, doesn't mean that it's not going to turn someone else into a zombie. This is another example of how people are different. Why is that so hard for many people to grasp? I've met individuals who can't get enough Maury Povich; yet if you forced me to watch that show, I might not ever talk to you again. We know people are different in their preferences; if they weren't, how would John Tesh have a fan base at all? Since people can have different tastes, doesn't it make sense that they could have different chemistry as well?

The Coalition for Health Education has an online university that teaches health care practitioners and anyone with a desire to learn about nutrition and many of the other topics I'm discussing in this book. They allow regular, non-professional people to take many of their courses, since many individuals just like to learn more about health. Some may want to gain more information to see if they might like to start a career as a health coach. In any case, they have a free course on pH that digs into this topic deeper than I cover it in this book. If the pH of the body interests you, this is an amazing free way to learn more. You can find these courses at www.CoalitionUniversity.org.

Imbalance - Tending to Acidosis

The physiology in a person with Acidosis problems expresses too much acid (or H+) in the bloodstream. One cause can be an imbalance in potassium, or an inability of the kidneys to properly excrete the acid and balance is lost. The breath rate in these individuals becomes accelerated because the kidneys, being unable to easily control the acid level in the bloodstream, can be helped by the lungs huffing off CO2, because CO2 acidifies the bloodstream. These individuals will normally have a short breath-holding time and a rapid breathing rate, exposing the fact that the kidneys are not having an easy time controlling the pH of the blood. This can be remedied (depending on the cause) by assisting the system to buffer the acids more effectively and excreting them. But this is not just a failure to excrete acids, it's a failure to buffer them. This helps us to understand why using foods or supplements in an effort to "alkalize" an individual can be so beneficial. This is how a pH guru can hit home runs with some people who will then think he is so brilliant. These people with the overly acid issues can really benefit by increasing the nutrients that can be used to buffer these acids. Even a broken clock is right twice a day.

An inability to properly digest protein can often be an issue in these cases since the biggest buffer of acids in the body is protein. Obviously, it is more profitable for the industry to sell green drinks and alkalizing supplements than it is to help people better digest their protein. Yet, in some cases, simply improving protein digestion can be a great step toward giving the body the tools it needs to buffer those acids on its own.

Possible symptoms that can show up with an Acid Imbalance:
- shortness of breath
- rapid heart rate
- allergies
- poor retention of important mineral nutrients
- fluid retention
- poor function of your kidneys, lungs, adrenal glands and many other organs and glands
- digestive issues

CHAPTER SEVEN

Digestion

Now, the mother of all chapters. Digestion is one of the most important aspects of health. I think it was Moses who once said, "He who doth not digest, doth not have good stuff," or something like that. I may be paraphrasing; I may have even added the word "digest" where it didn't belong and switched some other things around too, I'm not sure. The point is, digestion is crucial—and whether I said it or someone who you would have respected a lot more said it, I'm still going to talk about digestion a whole bunch.

This truly is the most paramount chapter of the book. As a matter of fact, if you read any of my other *Kick It in the Nuts* titles in the future, they will likely include a chapter on digestion. I'm even writing a fictional novel about a young boy who can't find his dog, and since digestion is so important, I'm thinking about including this chapter in that book as well. Digestive issues can rear their heads in an unlimited number of symptoms, conditions, diseases and even flat out crazy spells where you might think you're a humming bird. Most people think that if they stick food in the top end and something comes out of the bottom end, they must have digested it. That is not always the case. To fully break down the myths, explain the functions, and look at how digestion can relate to cramps, I have a lot to cover. It is my belief that this will be the most eye-opening chapter of *Kick Menstrual Cramps in the Nuts*.

137

Before I get to the mechanics of how digestion works, let's take a peek at why it is so important.

Losing Your Period And Pre-Menopausal Symptoms

To make a baby takes a lot of minerals and other types of nutrients. Believe it or not, babies aren't just delivered by a stork; it takes resources to build a baby just like it takes resources to build anything. Would you try to build a house without any building materials? Would you start construction without any wood, nails, bricks, concrete or whatever else you were going to build your house out of? Of course not. Your housewarming party would just be a bunch of people standing in your yard eating egg salad while they talked about how you've lost your marbles. Just as when building a house, you need resources if you want to make a cute little human.

When a woman has horribly low resources, Mother Nature will often protect the would-be mother from troublesome issues by turning off the woman's ability to have a baby... and the menstrual cycle stops until her resources come back up. But we often punch Mother Nature in the face and work around her by using pharmaceutical hormones that keep the cycle regular. One of the most common underlying causes for a woman to experience irregular periods, or to go months at a time without a period, is a lack of proper digestion. Digestion is what allows us to take the food we consume and turn it into life-sustaining resources. Once a woman can fully break down her food and pull the needed minerals out of what she's eating, her period commonly comes back. That's what we're doing when we digest. We're breaking down that food into elemental parts that can be used by the body. Believe it or not, the body cannot run on a peanut butter sandwich any more than your car can run on crude oil. It just won't work. However, what your body can do is break down that peanut butter sandwich into minerals, amino acids, fats and sugars and then use those nutrients. The body needs those nutrients. When digestion is not working properly and we can no longer break down our food enough to pull the required nutrients out of what we have eaten, systems begin to fail, just like your car would fail if it ran out of gas.

We are taught that menopause is all about these crazy hormonal changes that take place in a woman's body when she reaches a certain point in her life, as if there is this clock in her body that's been waiting fifty years to go off; and once it does, all hell breaks loose. Hormones run amok, the menstrual cycle begins to go haywire, and "Why does my face feel like I'm on fire for forty seconds at a time?" Many women are advised to start cramming hormones into their body in order to "correct" this hormonal imbalance that comes with age. Do you really think you can balance out your hormones better than Mother Nature? Why don't we ever stop to think that there might be a reason that these hormone levels are going crazy? Doesn't it make sense that, if the body is no longer receiving enough minerals and other nutrients it needs to function correctly, it might try to fix things on its own by raising hormone levels in a last-ditch effort to keep the body in a reproductive state? Once the body has tried every trick it has, the cycle will shut down and that individual will no longer have the ability to produce a child.

This can be viewed as a self-defense mechanism. If you've read some of my other books, you know there is a long list of symptoms and conditions that can result from a lack of resources: Depression, insomnia, mental disorder on top of mental disorder... the list goes on and on. If a woman with low resources has a baby and gives all of her resources to that baby, the mother is left with just enough to keep her alive. The baby basically stripped the mother of everything she was using to function. That's why postpartum depression is so common; the mother doesn't have the resources left to function properly and she feels depressed. To understand this better, read my upcoming book, *Kick Depression in the Nuts*. Until then, the contents of this section alone can help you see the multitude of troublesome issues that can develop from a lack of resources. To keep this from happening, the body shuts down the reproductive system when resources are low so the mother can just hang on to the small amount of resources she does have. Our bodies are quite genius.

Sex Is The Blossom Of Life

Look at it this way: sex is the blossom of life. Children don't reach puberty and gain the ability to reproduce until they are somewhere around the age of twelve to fourteen years old. (I think I was fourteen before I started seeing hair under my arms, but I had to color it in with my sister's mascara to really be able to see it.) Before children reach puberty, they are unable to reproduce. The digestive systems of children are not complete and fully functioning—at least, not to the point where they can produce another human. When the digestive system is complete, it can be said that the child has reached the "bloom of youth." If you say that to teenagers they will never stop making fun of you, but let's stick with this analogy anyway. Let's say there is a happy little tomato plant with the beginnings of a juicy red tomato just starting to blossom. However, what if this happy little plant falls on hard times, like a drought? (Insert evil music here... dun dun dun.) There is no water and no way for nutrients to make it up from the soil, so our poor little plant is basically starving. In order to survive, it will pull back the energy it was using to blossom that future juicy red tomato; instead it will use those resources to keep itself alive. That tiny little bud will fall off before it matures into a tomato and we will be sad because now our salsa is nothing but a bowl of chopped onions. Doesn't it make sense that the plant couldn't possibly bear fruit if it hardly had enough resources to survive?

When my colleagues and I work with women who have lost their cycles, possibly even for years, we often see their cycles return once they start to improve their digestive system. It's my experience that, when this happens, women are not pleased—but I am. I mean, this is really a trophy. The blossom reappeared on the plant and this is a prize worth cherishing. Since there is now

140

enough reserve energy in the system that the woman can again put forth a blossom, I know she really made her digestion come back. That's exciting to see. Don't you think it is beneficial for the body to have enough resources to function the way it is meant to? In the world today, people are going around saying, "Well, I've got all these hormonal problems." I am not saying that we don't have any legitimate hormonal problems today; we do. What I am advocating is to simply look first at digestion and see what's going on there before we blame the body because we have too much estrogen, or too little estrogen, or too much progesterone or too little progesterone. We should first look to bring back the vitality by improving digestion. The reason things are out of balance simply may be that the necessary resources are not there.

Sometimes digestion is only part of the problem. I can talk to clients and they will tell me, "Well, I think I need hormone replacement therapy." I can talk to them and ask questions like, "What time did you eat breakfast?" They'll say something like, "Oh, I just had some coffee, I really don't eat breakfast. I'm usually busy and don't eat until 2 o'clock." If I ask them when they eat again they'll say, "I usually eat around 7 o'clock at night, then I go to bed around eleven or twelve." If this sounds familiar to you, let me tell you what I tell them. If you have children and you send them to school without lunch money and no breakfast, and they are gone from 7am to 2 o'clock in the afternoon without eating, that could be 18 hours without food, depending on when they ate the night before. Child welfare will come and take your children away from you because that's flat out neglect. You wouldn't expect a child to excel with that type of neglect, so why would you expect a different outcome from your own body? In most cases, people who live this way don't really need hormone replacement therapy, they need breakfast. Yes, digestion is important and that's what I'm covering here, but how are you going to digest anything if you don't first insert it into your gullet?

141

How Digestion Works

It is very common for an individual to have poorly functioning digestion. Here's how it is designed to work:

When we eat, our stomachs make hydrochloric acid (HCL). Technically speaking, "HCl" is the correct capitalization because it is Hydrogen (H) and Chloride (Cl) on the periodic table. However, many writers and supplement labels use "HCL" because it is easier to read so I'll be following their lead. This stomach acid, as it is often called, has a pH of around 0.8. The pH scale goes from zero to fourteen. Zero means acidity to the max. Fourteen means alkalinity to the max.

When contents of the stomach (what we eat and drink) are mixed with this stomach acid, that combination will ideally have a pH between 2.0 and 3.0. The acidic product created by mixing stomach acid with the food you eat then goes into the duodenum (first ten inches of the small intestine). The other "half" of the digestive process comes from the bile that is produced by your liver. (I say "half of the digestive process" loosely because there are other factors that contribute to digestion that I cover later in this chapter. But for the most part, the main factors in digestion are the acid created in the stomach and the bile produced by the liver.) Between meals, bile is stored in the gallbladder where it is concentrated up to 18 times. When acid product from the stomach moves into the duodenum, bile from the gallbladder is dropped onto this acid product. In the same way that HCL is acidic, bile is alkaline (which is the opposite of acidic). Bile usually has a pH between 8.0 and 8.5. Since a pH of 7.0 is considered neutral, some may say that 8.5 is not that alkaline. But compared to a pH of 2.0 or 3.0, which is the contents coming from the stomach, this is a difference of over one hundred thousand times in the pH world.

That's like dropping baking soda onto vinegar, just like at least one 6th grader does every year when he makes his version of a volcano for his science fair project. In fact, you should try that now. You don't need to build the whole volcano, because let's face it, they might remove you from the board of directors if they find out you are building a fake volcano. What you can do is put a little bowl in your kitchen sink, put a couple teaspoons of baking soda in the bowl, and then slowly pour in a little vinegar. You'll hear a sizzle and see it start to foam up. C'mon, really do it! All the cool kids are doing it. It's a great visualization of what can happen when two substances with opposite pHs meet.

This is the magic of digestion. When the body drops bile (which also contains bicarb and enzymes from the pancreas) onto the contents that comes from the stomach, you get a sizzle, and this is what you're living on. You are living on this fast metabolic press that happens when the acid meets the alkalinity of the bile. This is what makes everything that was in the food break apart and become available for your body to use. Without this sizzle, foods you eat can't be assimilated. Nutrients and minerals can't be extracted and utilized by your body if this action is missing. That's why you hear so many people say, "Health is like a science fair project." Okay, I've never heard anyone say that, but if you don't have that sizzle in your digestion, you might as well be that 12-year-old holding the volcano with an "F" on it because the damn lava didn't come out. You've got to have the sizzle.

Therefore, in order for digestion to work properly, every step of that process has to be active. If there isn't enough stomach acid, there won't be that sizzle. If there isn't enough bile to drop down onto the food that was mixed with the stomach acid, there won't be that sizzle. So, instead of a sizzle, you get more of a fizzle and you may just break down a very small portion of your food, or your food will partially break down by processes of rotting and fermenting. This rotting and fermenting creates chemical reactions and gases that can cause bloating, burping, nausea, bad breath, upset stomach, and all kinds of other non-fun stuff. Have you ever been around someone who had breath that smelled like a garbage can? Most people look at bad breath as a dental hygiene

143

issue, and it can be; but more often than not it's a situation of, "I have food rotting in my stomach and intestines and the stench it creates is coming out of my mouth." Yes, I know you've met that guy.

This repulsive rotting of last night's dinner can also be the reason you don't feel like eating the next morning. Many of you, who I just yelled at about not eating breakfast, truly have no appetite when you wake up. Some people are even nauseous because last night's dinner still hasn't fully digested. It's just sitting there rotting, so of course they're not hungry. Their bodies are telling them, "Look, I haven't finished dealing with this garbage you sent down here last night, please don't dump anything else on top of it." By improving digestion, your morning appetite can improve as well.

More On HCL

We all know the body makes stomach acid. But when we hear about stomach acid, it's usually how people have "too much" acid and that's why they are dealing with heartburn or acid reflux issues. There is a lot of brilliant marketing that goes on by the pharmaceutical companies when it comes to stomach acid and why it might be a good idea to turn acid off, and I believe it the same way I believe that a mime is a talented artist. In chapter eight, I explain why people really get heartburn and reflux, but let's first look at why "turning off" your stomach acid with these drugs is one of the worst possible things you can do for your long-term health.

Hydrochloric acid (HCL) is the protector of the human body. Let's say you are eating at the buffet and you're taking in viruses, bacteria, and microorganisms because you scoop up the salad the kids sneezed on a few minutes earlier. While you eat from this salad bar, you are taking in all this filth and you are eating undercooked hamburger and chicken drummettes that were dropped on the floor. The truth is you don't really know what

144

you are getting. Keep in mind that I worked at a salad bar when I was a kid and my only rule was that being funny in front of the cute waitresses was far more important to me than delivering clean, sanitary food to all the red-neck patrons that came in on coupon night. Your food doesn't even need to be dropped on the floor by a zit-faced high school kid to have bacteria or other little creatures on it. Even the food you clean and prepare at home can have some little ninja-like varmints that make it through the cleaning process. (Varmints! 500 points to me for fitting in a Yosemite Sam reference.)

That's where HCL becomes such a hero. Anything that comes into YOU (any microorganisms, bacteria, or other types of bad guys) are going to die in an acid bath. That stomach acid is the protector of the mechanism that is YOU. The hydrochloric acid function of the stomach is your knight in very disgusting armor. When you take a drug that turns that barrier off, you're opening the door to anybody that wants to come in and raid the pantry (you are the pantry in this scenario). That's why two people can eat the same meal and one will get food poisoning and have projectile fluids coming out of both ends and the other person will just say, "The fish didn't taste right, did it? Oh, and sorry about your luck." One person had the proper level of stomach acid to kill whatever little bastards were still living on that fish and the other person is praying to the porcelain god, vowing to never eat seafood again.

Why doesn't ketchup spoil on the restaurant table? I mean, it's been sitting there for a month and it didn't turn white with bacteria? It is often said that no bacteria can grow in a terrain that has a pH below 4.5. It is kind of a canning industry standard, loosely speaking, that pickles and ketchup must have a pH under 4.5. That's because botulism doesn't grow in a pH under 4.5 and a lot of other bacteria have a difficult time growing in an environment where the pH is below 4.5 as well. Of course apple cider vinegar is made from bacteria and that's usually running a pH around 3. So, there are bacteria that do live down in a low pH range, but most of them are not that pathogenic, which is why humans can drink apple cider vinegar and it can have health benefits for some people—not all people, but some.

The point is, you want that acid function to be in the stomach because it is the gatekeeper. It's the lock that keeps all the hoodlums out. I don't want you to think that taking medication for acid reflux or heartburn is the only reason a person may lose that acid function. There are many ways a person can produce less than the proper levels of acid. It is already known that acid levels can be reduced by using drugs that are intended for that purpose, but it needs to be understood how this can turn into an endless pattern that may turn off digestion for decades.

Minerals And HCL

Once digestion is interrupted for an extended period of time, this vicious cycle can continue for a lifetime. In order for your body to pull the minerals out of the food you eat, your digestion must be working properly. You must be producing enough HCL and you must have the proper bile flow to get that sizzle that pulls the minerals out of your food. The dilemma is, the body needs certain minerals in order to make HCL. Do people lack the ability to digest because they don't have the mineral to make HCL, or do they lack the mineral to make HCL because they don't have the ability to digest? Does it matter? Either way, these people are screwed and need to find a way to break this vicious cycle.

Chloride and zinc are both important components when it comes to making HCL and I talk about ways to boost your levels, and even kick-start the system with HCL supplementation, in chapter twelve when I cover digestive supplements. If you need a preview for the plan now, just know that if you can supply your body with HCL through supplementation, while you also increase specific minerals in the system through supplementation, you can manufacture good digestion. Once you do this, your body will have all it needs to begin creating its own HCL and the supplementation will no longer be needed. However, there is a very specific plan that should be followed when trying to improve HCL production, so be sure you fully understand it before you start to use any type of HCL supplement. Otherwise, you will give yourself a duodenal ulcer or you'll feel like you have crazy heartburn. So, simma down and wait until you've read through chapter twelve before you jump into any HCL efforts. You first need to figure out if HCL is even right for you. Remember, don't just go off of symptoms. You need to understand where your chemistry is. If you only learn one thing from this book, I want that one thing to be this: If you use a supplement because all the cool kids are using it, you're going to get yourself into trouble.

H. Pylori

It is believed that the most common cause of lowered stomach acidity is chronic infection by Helicobacter pylori (H. pylori). This organism is the most recurrent bacterial pathogen in humans and can infect the body for decades without creating any direct, flu-like symptoms. H. pylori are resistant to most antibiotics and can even avoid being wiped out by stomach acid. It is true that stomach acid must be temporarily low in order for H. pylori to infect; but once they are in, when stomach acid rises back to the proper level, H. pylori can migrate below the mucous layer in the stomach and protect themselves from the acid.

Once colonized, H. pylori create ammonia as a waste product. Ammonia is alkaline and can reduce the acidity of the stomach, therefore making the stomach a more hospitable home for the bacteria. It has also been shown that chronic H. pylori infection can result in the atrophy of the stomach's functional components that produce HCL. Since studies have shown that H. pylori eats hydrogen, and hydrogen is needed to produce HCL, many believe that the functional components are "not working" because all the hydrogen has been scarfed up by the H. pylori. By "turning off" the acid production, so to speak, H. pylori has now made your stomach a very happy party place, not only for H. pylori, but also for just about any bad guys that show up for the kegger they are throwing this Friday night. And to bacteria, every night is Friday night.

Some studies have shown that an individual who eradicates a chronic H. pylori infection may not fully recover the stomach's acid producing function for twelve months or more after the bacteria have been wiped out. It is still unclear exactly how H. pylori turns off acid production, but it is clear that H. pylori have the ability to do so. I go over some methods to shut down H. pylori's party in chapter twelve when I cover digestive supplements, but certainly removing an H. pylori infection would be a key step in correcting any digestive issues.

CHAPTER EIGHT

Digestion Gone Wild

Reflux, Heartburn And GERD

Now that you understand the benefits of both acid production and bile flow working correctly, let's talk about some issues that can pop up when one side is not working optimally. I promised earlier that I would explain the fiction that is the billion dollar industry of reflux, heartburn, and GERD (gastroesophageal reflux disease). The marketing surrounding this issue may mislead an individual more than just about any other current health information out there. First of all, there are many different causes of reflux; but very few cases, if any, are actually caused by "too much acid," as advertisers explain when marketing their products.

At the bottom of your esophagus, there is a little valve called an LES, or lower esophageal sphincter. This valve opens to let food enter the stomach and then it closes, so that the food doesn't go back up your esophagus and burn you. Sometimes, people have a small hiatal hernia where part of the stomach is pulled up into the diaphragm. This can keep that valve from closing and can result in an acid reflux problem. That is one possibility.

However, the most common cause of reflux problems involves the acid level of the stomach. The LES is actually HCL sensitive, meaning that when the stomach makes enough HCL, it activates that valve to close so digesting food doesn't reflux back up. I've already mentioned that some people don't make enough HCL on their own. So doesn't it make sense that, if there isn't enough HCL in the stomach to trigger the valve, the valve would stay open and they would get reflux? People aren't having reflux because of too much acid; they're having reflux because there is not enough acid.

Pharmaceutical companies sell us drugs that turn the acid off, so that when we experience reflux, we can't feel the burning and we assume the originating issue has been dealt with. The problem with that is twofold. First, the stomach also contains digestive enzymes that can come back up with reflux. These digestive enzymes are made to break down protein. What is the esophagus made of? Yes, protein. Therefore, using these drugs stops the burning sensation, but it doesn't stop the damage that reflux can cause. The second problem created by turning off the acid is... you just turned off the acid. I've already covered how important your stomach acid is, how it is the safety barrier for your entire body and how it's an ignorant idea to turn it off. So, why do you want to be misled by an ignorant person?

When you hear about a drug being a proton pump inhibitor (PPI), this refers to the hydrogen proton pump in the human body. These drugs restrict the body from producing hydrogen. Hydrogen is required for the body to make its own HCL, so by turning off the hydrogen, you turn off the acid. Not only are the proton-pump-inhibitor-type drugs another punch in the mouth to your liver (I already discussed how all drugs work by overwhelming the liver enough to be able to stay in the system and do their job), they also turn off your digestion. Now, any food you eat not only doesn't nourish your body like it is intended to, but also this undigested, rotting, fermenting food becomes another problem for your body to try to remove or to store in fat cells. Pretty good little pill, huh?

To reduce reflux, nine out of ten reflux sufferers can actually *increase* the amount of stomach acid they have which will trigger the LES to close so they no longer experience reflux. This also allows the body to fully break down its food, pull out the minerals and then use those minerals to make the proper amount of stomach acid. Look forward to reading more about how to improve these issues in *Kick Reflux, Heartburn & GERD in the Nuts,* but I talk about specifics on how to increase stomach acid in chapter twelve. First, it's a good idea to figure out if you're a person who could benefit from more stomach acid, so don't get ahead of me.

Crohns, Colitis, And IBS

What about the other end of digestion? What about the bile side of the action? If bile is not flowing well enough to neutralize the acid product coming from the stomach, now there is acid going through the intestines. And why does the stomach make acid? The primary job of stomach acid is digesting protein. It's the hydrochloric acid that breaks down food and allows protein to become accessible to the body. Think about it; if you don't neutralize that acid, what do you think it's going to do to your intestines? Your intestines are made out of protein, just like your esophagus. How about that? Does anybody you know have symptoms that were diagnosed as IBS, Crohns, or Colitis? Don't you think this could just be the acid that has been produced in the stomach, that has not been neutralized sufficiently in the duodenum by the proper amount of alkaline bile? Now this acid product goes through the intestines like "Zingo!" Why? Because the acidity of this product is making the intestines burn and the body is going to respond to this acidity and march that product right through the person in a big damn hurry. With this understanding, doesn't it make sense that it comes shooting out the back door in such a rush?

Beyond that, sodium likes to follow chloride. Water likes to follow sodium. So there's also going to be sodium that is attracted to this chloride in the hydrochloric acid (the hydrochloric acid that didn't get neutralized). Then more water will go to the bowels since chloride from HCL that has not been neutralized will draw the sodium with its water into the bowel. It would be like Justin Beiber showing up to your cookout because he wanted a hot dog. Not only would you have one less hot dog, you would also have a yard filled with thousands of screaming little girls. The good news is, the water rushing to this guy's bowels will help dilute this acid product that is burning the intestinal walls. The bad news is, he just crapped his pants. This guy is going to have diarrhea and he is going to wonder why, when he sits on the John, it's like he was shot from rockets. It's because his body is saying, "Get this acid product that is burning the daylights out of my little intestines out of here!"

Probiotics and gut flora are a hot topic these days. The people that experience these diarrhea-type issues need help in this arena because that un-neutralized acid scorching through their intestines just fried their gut flora. The terrain needs to be right for gut flora to flourish. As you can imagine, the towering inferno from hell is not the right terrain. This is a very vague explanation, and you will better understand this scenario when I release *Kick Crohns, Colitis, & IBS in the Nuts,* but it's a great visualization to help explain the balance that is required in order for digestion to function correctly. Both ends of the process are important. It's clear that trouble arises when one side or the other isn't holding up its end of the bargain.

Let's Talk Crap

There are two types of people in this world. There are stargazers and there are stoolgazers, and the stoolgazers fair better. There is a lot that can be learned from our poop—specifically, how our bodies are operating, and especially how well our digestion is working. If you understand what to look for, it's almost as good as if Mr. Hankey showed up in your toilet every day and told you

152

about what was going on in your digestive system. (For anyone who has never seen *South Park*, Mr. Hankey is a talking poop.)

Stool often moves at its level of acidity. As I talked about in the previous section, stool can move too quickly and be too loose when it is too acidic. Not only does this burn the intestines, but also, if the stool is moving too quickly, the body doesn't get the opportunity to absorb as many nutrients as it should. If stool is not acidic enough, it can move too slowly and even lead to constipation. This is not ideal either because toxins that the body was trying to remove can be re-absorbed and then need to be filtered out again, which can overwhelm a hard-working liver. Just don't jump to conclusions and think that this is your answer if you've been dealing with chronic constipation issues. This lack of acid is only one cause of constipation and is not always a factor in every constipation case. You'll find more answers in *Kick Constipation in the Nuts* (coming soon); but if you do improve your digestion with the guidelines I lay out in this book, and your constipation issues improve, you'll know that you've likely found the main cause.

If you see food in your stool, that's a screaming sign that you're not digesting well. If you eat salad and poop salad, guess what... you didn't break down that salad. Your stool should come out solid, formed, darker than the color of cardboard, and you shouldn't be able to sift through and recognize what you ate (I really hope you don't sift through it). If you don't have the award-winning poop that I just described, it's time to give your digestion some attention. So, be a stoolgazer, find out what's going on at the south gate. When you see a full buffet coming out down there, then you know there is not enough hydrochloric acid and some steps need to be taken. I talk more about those steps in chapter twelve.

I asked one low-HCL client if when he eats salad he poops salad. He said "No I don't. When I eat salad, I poop coleslaw."

Stool color is another great indicator. If your stool is lighter than the color of cardboard, that's an indication that bile is not flowing very well. Bile is dark green and that is what makes stool a darker color. If your stool comes out dark green, it's possible that your bile is flowing well, but you don't have enough acid to mix with the bile and create that sizzle. If your stool color presents more variations of the rainbow, that's not great either. If you drink fourteen purple Slurpees and your poop comes out purple, that's just an indication that you need to spend less time shopping at the 7-11. But if color varies while eating normal foods, there are likely issues. If it's light sometimes and dark others, you're probably not emulsifying your fats correctly and the color is varying according to how much fat you ate. If you eat a big plate of vegetables and your stool is green, when it normally isn't, odds are you're not breaking down those vegetables well enough. Dark brown is what you're shooting for. C'mon, you can do it. Poop brown. (After writing that paragraph, I think "purple Slurpee" might be my new favorite phrase. When I leave the house today I'm going to use it when I greet the first few people I see. I feel like it will confuse them to the point where a response will be impossible. You can try it too. "What's up, purple Slurpee?")

Burping, Bloating And Passing Gas

Here is a more detailed explanation of the snippet in chapter five. Here's the ultimate question to figure out if you're really bloating. (This question only works for women because men are way too oblivious of their bodies to get this one.) Are your clothes tighter in the evening when you take them off than in the morning when you put them on? If you so much as have to think about it, you're probably not bloating, because a woman knows. She will say, "Yeah, they are tighter when I take them off." She knows, and if they are tighter, she is bloating. So, if the acid product in the stomach is not sufficient then people are going to grow bacteria in their tummies. When they grow bacteria in their tummies, they are going to produce gas. It is the same as making beer or wine or champagne or root beer; all of these things are fermented. When you ferment, you are going to get gas and the gas is going to bloat. Some people may feel very bloated, while others may experience more burping.

When I say burping, I don't mean these huge belches. That may be the case with you, but that's not really what I'm talking about. Just little burps that are hardly even noticeable are usually a good sign that the stomach is not acidic enough. I see a lot of people who don't even realize that they're burping after their meals. Once I ask them, they come back later and say, "Hey, ya know what, I am burping after my meals and I never even noticed." Now, it's your turn to pay attention and see if you're burping too. Whether you're burping because of the gas created by undigested food rotting and fermenting, or the gases created by bacteria that are living in your stomach, or a combination of both, taking stock of what is going on with your body is the first step to making any improvements.

People think, "Everyone passes gas, what's the big deal?" The problem is most adults don't have their digestion working correctly anymore and that is why gas is so common. If you're passing gas, it's usually because your bile isn't flowing well enough. If your bile isn't dropping into the duodenum to meet the acid product from the stomach, you're not digesting properly.

Digestive Enzymes

Enzymes are another factor that play into the digestive process. All living foods are intended to contain enzymes that actually help you digest that food better. Be that as it may, with today's despicable farming methods, even many raw foods do not contain the needed enzymes to correctly digest those foods. On top of that, any time food is processed or heated over 118 degrees (pretty much any time you cook food), the enzymes are killed and you will not get the full benefit from that food. In order to fully break down the food you eat, you can supplement enzymes with your food. As we age, the body's stockpile of usable enzymes diminishes. People over thirty should be supplementing enzymes with their food. If you don't supply your body with the enzymes it needs, your body steals enzymes intended for repair processes and turns them into digestive enzymes, leaving fewer repair-enzymes for their intended use.

With certain imbalances, TOO MANY enzymes can facilitate deterioration. So, you want to take just enough to help you digest your food. Many enzyme companies promote taking unlimited enzymes but that is not recommended with some imbalances.

Conquering Our Food - Food Allergies

When you eat a salami sandwich (and no, I'm not recommending that you eat a salami sandwich... it's just fun to say salami sandwich), the goal is to conquer that sandwich instead of having it carry you off captive. Food allergies are a very hot topic these days and people come to me all the time and tell me about the testing they had done for food allergies. They tell me their tests showed they're allergic to nuts, dairy, wheat, gluten, soy, pork, turkey jerky, the board game Parcheesi, and Lou Diamond Phillips. Well, at what point does this person have to leave Earth in order to eat lunch? He's been told that he's allergic to just about everything on the planet. If you get to the point where you can only eat things that resemble Al Roker, it might be time to understand food allergies.

You may have already come across some of the rules or diets that are out there to help those with food sensitivities. There are gluten-free diets, blood-type diets, food-combining diets, raw-food diets, this list could keep going all the way down to the "*Saved by the Bell*, Zack & Kelly" diet. Most of these diets can actually benefit some individuals, but many people who need to employ a diet like this in order to feel better could find similar relief by correcting any digestive issues they may be experiencing. Once you can fully digest what you're eating, the need to complete the "Screech-free" phase of the Zack & Kelly diet becomes obsolete.

The point is, let's conquer what we eat. A carrot is not supposed to carry us off captive. We are to dominate the carrot; the carrot is not to dominate us. You ate it, you chewed it, it's yours. You're going to make YOU out of it. The chemistry of life is on this planet for you to take advantage of; but if you don't have digestion, you can't even take a supplement and have it work. People have all these stories of this food is good for you and that food is good for you. Hey, if you can't digest it, there is no food good for you. All that information is baloney, because without digestion it's good for no one.

So, what are all of these theories about food based on? There are so many books and diets and "gurus" out there it's enough to make you lose your appetite, even if you did know what you were supposed to eat. So, who's right? Do I eat for my blood type? Do I alkalize? Do I avoid carbs? Do I eat whatever I want as long as it starts with the letter "B"? Who's right? Well, I don't know. Whose research was everybody using as a basis for fact when they came up with these diets? Maybe most of the test subjects they used did, indeed, thrive on the ice cream sandwich diet. But, if you're interested in how the human body works, which I know I am, you first need to know how that particular human's digestion is functioning. If digestion is not so great, there is no diet that will fix all that person's woes.

This is the reason juicing has become so popular. Many fancy-pants gurus advocate buying these blenders that cost as much as a car and can liquefy your iPhone in thirty seconds. They tell us that we need to liquefy our food or we can't pull the nutrients out. And they're right, if you're a person with horrible digestion. That's why so many people feel better when they start to juice— they're actually getting some nutrients into the system. I do find that these juicing maniacs get a little upset when they learn that simply fixing their digestion can give them the same benefit. "You mean it was unnecessary for me to blend my turkey meatloaf and brussels sprouts and drink it through a straw?"

Let me get back to the point and break down these food allergies a little bit. Enzymes can play a factor in food sensitivities. If people don't have the correct enzymes to break down a specific type of food, that food can give them trouble. Take dairy for example. Many cases of lactose intolerance are just situations where people are lacking the enzyme lactase. If they supplement this enzyme, they may see improvement with their intolerance. I talked about enzymes a little bit in this chapter, and I cover them more in chapter twelve when I get into digestive supplements; but most adults in this day and age should be supplementing enzymes with their food.

The main cause for food allergies, however, normally has more to do with improper digestion than a lack of enzymes. I talked earlier about how your body can't use a peanut butter sandwich until that sandwich has been broken down into elemental nutrients. This same understanding is used when looking at food allergies. Once you break down that peanut butter sandwich, it's no longer a peanut butter sandwich. Instead, it is now minerals, fats, amino acids—the things your body needs—and now they all have a little picture of your face on them because they are going to become a part of you. As these nutrients move through your body, the bodily systems wave and smile as they pass with that picture of your face on them. These nutrients are welcome and the body is excited to see them.

However, if you never break down that peanut butter sandwich because your digestion is not working properly, that food still has its own identity since it was never conquered. That identity says, "Hi, I'm a peanut butter sandwich." Well, there is no use for a "peanut butter sandwich" in the body. The body can only use the nutrients that are pulled out of that peanut butter sandwich once it has been broken down by a functioning digestive system. If this peanut butter sandwich enters the system and still has its own identity, it is looked upon by the body as an invader and will be attacked and removed. A peanut butter sandwich is not going to have a picture of your face on it as it moves through the system. For this reason, everyone is going to run and scream and sound the alarms. As your immune system creates antibodies to deal with this invader, an imprint of those antibodies is saved in the "security files." Now, the next time you eat a peanut butter sandwich, all hell breaks loose as the system comes down hard on this "invader" and you can feel an "allergic response." And why wouldn't you? Your body just went to war against a peanut butter sandwich for cryin' out loud. You're not supposed to be trying to digest a peanut butter sandwich in your bloodstream using your immune system.

PLEASE NOTE: This is not to say that someone with a peanut allergy or something as severe and life-threatening as that should not take it seriously. They absolutely should. That is not what I'm talking about here. Most of those individuals were born with an allergy like that. I'm talking about sensitivities that people have developed in their life due to an inability to digest, or conquer, their food.

Birth Control Medications

Birth control medications work because they close off the fallopian tubes, preventing the eggs from dropping. Now the woman can't get pregnant, so it works. The problem is, the mechanism in the drug can't tell the difference between a fallopian tube and a gallbladder tube, so it can close the latter off as well. The level at which the gallbladder tube is closed can vary from woman to woman. If the gallbladder tube is shut, bile can't flow correctly and I've already covered how much that can blow.

When bile can't flow correctly, you can't properly digest your food and pull the needed minerals and nutrients out of what you're eating. You may also get nauseous because bile is the main method that the body uses to remove toxins out the south gate (bowels). If your bile flow reduces because of birth control meds, those toxins can build up and you can experience nausea. It's your body's way of telling you, "Look, we can't handle the food you've put in here, do you really need to keep adding more?"

In addition to turning off the body's main path of junk removal, birth control medications are a synthetic drug. In order for the dose to stay in the body long enough to do its job, it has to be a dose high enough to overwhelm the liver. Otherwise, the liver would just remove it from the body. So, any drug can't work unless it first punches your liver in the mouth. Now, the drug occupies the liver and the liver can't do its normal job of removing toxins. As the toxins get backed up, you get nauseous or you can gain weight since your body is forced to store those toxins in fat cells.

Birth control meds are also believed to kill all, or most of, your intestinal flora. If birth control medication stops a woman's bile from flowing correctly, there is nothing to cool off the acid product coming from the stomach and the intestinal flora can burn up. Without the beneficial bacteria, bad guys start to take over, creating an overgrowth of harmful bacteria and yeast, like candida.

Just in case you didn't catch my drift here, birth control medication can be one of the worst things a woman can do if she wants to have a healthy body. I realize pregnancy has the potential to wreak havoc on the body as well; at least with pregnancy, 10 years later you have someone to take out your trash for you. However, there is a freedom of choice in these matters, and there are birth control options available that will allow you to continue digesting your food properly.

Gallbladder Removal/Gallstones/Olive Oil-Lemon Drink

When I see a client with health issue after health issue, one of my first questions is, "Do you still have your gallbladder?" Doctors are taught that the gallbladder really doesn't do anything anyway; so, if there are stones or blockages, why not just yank it out? The problem is that your gallbladder is where your body stores bile, and without the proper amount of bile, you can't digest your food completely. The gallbladder also concentrates the bile and makes it stronger, so that when its alkalinity drops down on the acid product from the stomach, there is a good digestive sizzle. You've already learned how proper digestion is needed to obtain nutrients from your food. Eventually, without proper digestion, all the mineral and nutrient deficiencies will cause problems and even imbalances. The majority of health issues lead back to digestion in one way or another. You can digest food correctly only if you have enough acid in your stomach, enough bile from the gallbladder, and bicarb and enzymes from the pancreas dropping down into your duodenum. Without a gallbladder there is no bile storage, so you rarely have enough bile.

The digestive system is a crazy, complex, miraculous machine. Every aspect of this machine works together with the rest of the digestive process. With so many bits and pieces at play, the system is vulnerable to problems that would cause it to function below par. Do you really think a system will work the way it is meant to if you take out part of it (i.e. the gallbladder) and chuck it in the garbage? When any part of the digestive process is not functioning, troubles can show up for months, decades, or even a lifetime. You may not even know you're having digestive concerns because you feel okay when you eat (or you've forgotten what it feels like to feel good). But the lack of nutrients coming into the system, which can be created by a lack of digestion, is always going to come back to bite you in the ass. They may even literally bite you in the ass. (That was a parasite joke for those who didn't keep up.)

There is one technique that can simulate bile production from the gallbladder. Many people who have lost their gallbladder use this technique with success to improve their digestion. You can buy ox bile supplements in most health food stores. However, remember that bile is alkaline. If you take an ox bile product with your food, you're going to neutralize your stomach acid while it's still in your stomach. That's not fun. The trick is to take the ox bile product about two hours after a meal, or at least an hour before a meal. I like the hour before a meal best, but it can be difficult to remember that all the time. By moving that bile through your intestines between your meals, you can neutralize the acid product coming from your stomach and almost simulate the sizzle that all the cool kids have in their digestion. This ox bile really isn't going to work as well as true digestion, but without a gallbladder, this ox bile schedule can be one of the most effective options for any type of improvement.

Many people who have had their gallbladder removed will eventually end up with some type of loose stool issue. Since there isn't enough bile storage to neutralize the acid coming from the stomach, that acid just keeps trucking through the intestinal tract. The hitch is that this issue usually arises months or even years after they've had their gallbladder removed, so they never connect the two events. Using an ox bile product (as I described in the previous paragraph) is the most effective method I know to improve or prevent these loose stool issues, outside of buying a used gallbladder from someone at a garage sale (though I'm not sure how that would work with all the haggling that goes on at garage sales).

If you have gallstones and you're thinking about having your gallbladder removed, you might want to try smashing yourself in the face with a hammer instead. You may indeed prefer a nice hammer smashing over some of the troubles I have seen from

162

people who have had their gallbladder removed. There are things you can do to improve your gallbladder function and help soften those gallstones without cutting out the whole package. If someone told you that your big toe needed to be removed, you would make sure he knew what he was talking about; you would also be careful that you did not get a "second opinion" from some crony of the guy who gave you the first opinion. We know that because of gangrene or something very grievous, some big toes do need to be removed. But if you went into the doctor's office with toenail fungus and the doctor said the answer was to cut off your toe, you would probably find somebody else to help you. It seems a person would value his gallbladder at least as much as his big toe. I think internal organs generally eclipse appendages in value, but that's just me. If doctors were educated on how digestion really works, it would eliminate the billion dollar industry of antacids and acid-stopping drugs. Since doctors are not educated on how digestion works, doesn't it make sense that they view the gallbladder as if it were a disposable Ziploc baggie that can just be dumped in the trash?

There is an old-school remedy for a gallbladder attack that still holds true today. They even used to put this remedy right on the label of every carton of Epsom salt. The label said, "Take 4 tsp. of Epsom salt mixed in warm water." This will clear most gallbladder attacks because it can squirt the bile through and clear out the blockage. Be warned that this little trick can give you some crazy diarrhea since Epsom salt is magnesium sulfate. Both magnesium and sulfur products can push more water to the bowels, so a large dose of magnesium sulfate can create a bit of a show shooting out the back door. But an episode of diarrhea beats a lifetime of diarrhea every time. You would still need to do the work to get your bile to flow better so you can soften up those stones and keep more stones from forming, but this is a great little trick that has worked for over a hundred years for those suffering from gallbladder attacks. I talk more about how to thin your bile and get it flowing better in chapter twelve.

There are some great recipes on the Internet for olive oil and lemon drinks that can help clear out a gallbladder. However, if you do any cleanses like this that can also clear out a liver, and your bile isn't flowing well, you're just dumping all these toxins into the body while the body has no way to remove them. This can trigger some crazy rashes as a result of the body trying to push junk out through the skin, or you can really overload and hurt your kidneys as they try to handle the whole load. With this in mind, be sure you learn how to thin your bile and get it flowing better with specific beet leaf products before you try any of those liver/gallbladder-type cleanses. They can bring about some big trouble if you don't. Are you listening to me right now? This is important, so don't ignore what I'm saying and go straight for a heavy duty liver cleanse without first addressing your bile flow with the beet leaf products described in chapter twelve. Man, you should really be excited about chapter twelve by now. I can't shut up about it.

Liver Function

I'm going to include some thoughts about liver function in this digestion chapter because proper bile flow is such a vital part of how effectively your liver is taking care of business. I say this a lot, and I'll probably say it three or four more times in this book, but in my opinion, the two most important factors for good health are digestion and liver function. I'm not trying to say that if people have a horrific imbalance in need of attention, or an extra limb growing out of the side of their head, that they first need to correct liver function. I'm just speaking generally when I say that the liver's ability to handle its affairs is a super big deal.

I've covered a multitude of factors that can reduce a liver's performance: Almost any medication, a lack of bile flow, bringing in more junk than the liver can remove, etc. Any of these things can trouble a liver; and if the liver isn't working optimally, eventually your body won't be working optimally either. Think of your liver like a huge ventilation fan that can clear smoke out of a kitchen or entire house. Growing up as a kid, my family lived in a big yellow two-story house. In the living room, just outside of the bathroom, was a huge ventilation fan that was built into the ceiling. It had a metal shutter-like covering that would open when the fan was on and then close when you turned off the fan. This prevented all the freaky, Floridian bugs from flying into the house when the gusting wind wasn't cranking from the fan blades.

My Mom had a friend who would come over to the house and smoke in the living room. Even at twelve years old, I hated cigarette smoke and didn't want to smell it in my house any more than I wanted to miss an episode of *The Muppet Show*. "Animal" was a bad ass drummer with serious skills and I just knew we would share a two set-up drum solo some day. Whenever my Mom's friend, Margaret, was over for a visit, I would turn on this huge fan and immediately it would suck all the smoke out of the house, as if it never existed. It's not that the house wasn't big enough to hold Margaret and myself at the same time, it was just too disgusting when that fan wasn't on.

This is similar to how your liver works. To say that your body can't handle a few toxins coming in is far from true. The liver is your body's massive ventilation fan. As junk comes in, the liver moves it out to keep the system clean and operating smoothly. I came home from school one day in a thunderstorm to find that our electricity was out. There was Margaret sitting on the couch. I could barely make out her beady little eyes through all the smoke, but I knew it was her. I immediately turned around to leave the house and my Mom asked where I was going. "Out to get struck by lightning," I said. I guess I was a jackass when I was a kid too. In the same way I was too miserable to exist in that house without the fan, you might be too miserable in your life without your liver working properly.

The ability for that fan to act like the "liver" of my house wasn't even its best feature. Remember those tall, round white hampers found in every family's laundry room in 1982? They were three feet tall and just wide enough to fit a person. This fan was so strong that when you turned it on, you could flip that hamper upside down and stick the bottom to the grate of the fan and the power of the wind would hold it there. The switch that turned it off was across the room, so anytime my little sister would go into the bathroom I would stick the hamper to the fan grate to set my trap. As she came out of the bathroom, I would flip off the fan and the hamper would fall down and slide over her unsuspecting little head and body. It was right out of a Bugs Bunny cartoon. The hamper was just long enough that it would pin her arms down and she would have no choice but to bounce off the living room furniture until she fell over and could finally wiggle out of the bottom. Yeah, she didn't like that so much.

You'll have a hard time torturing your little sister with your liver, but at least this helps explain how a properly working liver can be as effective as a properly working ventilation fan. After all the medical doctors had their way with me, and my liver was trashed from all the drugs I was taking, it was tough to even walk by some substances, much less take them into my body. When the liver is overwhelmed and can't handle the current load that it's already dealing with, it can be arduous for people to find foods they can eat without feeling miserable. There were only three or four very clean foods I could eat without feeling horrible because my body couldn't deal with the chemicals and preservatives found in most foods. Now that I have improved my liver function, those things don't bother me because my body can handle the trouble and my liver can remove those substances.

CHAPTER NINE

Other Factors With Cramps

Remember, there is no single cause for menstrual cramps. For most who suffer from cramps, the tissue calcium deficiency issue that I've been talking about throughout this book is a major player. In this section, I elaborate on that idea and also delve into other factors that may be contributing to your cramps. Furthermore, I'm hoping you'll find that this information may be beneficial to your health in general, even after your cramps disappear.

Chocolate, etc.

In chapter two I talked to you a little bit about vitamin D. I described how vitamin D can pull calcium out of the tissues and hold it in the bloodstream, reducing the amount of calcium that is at the tissue level. You certainly remember how that is a bad thing since it is often a deficiency of calcium at the tissue level that can intensify cramps. As soon as you learned all of this, you probably threw your vitamin D in the garbage or gave it to someone you don't like. I applaud your decision, but now we need to discuss something else that can mimic the result vitamin D can create when it comes to cramps. I know you're getting nervous right now, and yes, you're going to want to punch me in the head, but let's be strong together and just rip the Band-Aid off quickly. It's sugar.

Sugar, chocolate, complex carbs, all those things you crave—and crave even more around your period—are all contributing to your cramps. I know the cravings are crazy and I'm going to teach you why, and even how to get rid of them, so please put down the lighter if you are reading a printed version of this book. I always find it funny when clients think that I make the rules for what they can and cannot eat if they want to improve their cramps, as if I had that type of power over somebody. I don't make up the rules. I'm not the guy who decides how your body works, I just deliver the news and it's up to you how you want to use that information. Don't try to bargain with me and ask, "What if I tell ten friends to buy your book? Then, can I eat a Twix bar before bed every night?" It doesn't work that way. Do you really think that if I give you my blessing to eat a candy bar every night, that's going to reduce the amount of trouble that junk food is going to cause, just because I endorsed it? Do you really think I have the ability to change how science works? I am not equipped with that superpower—and if I were, that would be the geekiest superpower ever. I can only teach you how to reduce those cravings if you have them. Before I talk about how to improve this issue, let me first explain why these foods are a contributing factor with cramps.

Calcium tends to follow sugar. That was pretty simple. I've already gone over how, for most women who suffer from cramps, those cramps get worse when there is not enough calcium at the tissue level. Picture it this way... sugar comes into the system and all the calcium in the tissues looks at that sugar like it's an ice cream truck driving through the neighborhood. The calcium says, "Let's chase that ice cream truck," and it leaves the tissue, where it is meant to be, and follows the sugar into the bloodstream. Now the bloodstream is filled with sugar first and then calcium. Thicker blood results in your feeling great. However, your tissues have now been stripped of calcium and the troubles that are going to come next can include cramps, frequent viruses, charley horses, and more. The result can be different for every person, but an increase in severe cramps seems to be the most common result.

"But I read that dark chocolate is actually good for me." Yes, I understand that, but now you're reading this: Dark chocolate is not actually good for you. Dark chocolate does contain flavonoids and antioxidants that could be beneficial for some people, but it also contains enough sugar to cancel out any benefits those "healthy factors" would bring. If you were to use those nutrients on their own, yes they could be beneficial. But, to say that dark chocolate is actually healthy is like saying that broccoli dipped in rat poison is good for you because it's broccoli. Is chocolate a better choice than a deep fried pastry stuffed with amphetamines? Yes, it is. But that doesn't mean it's good for you. There are raw forms of chocolate, like raw cacao, that contain far less sugar; but these raw forms of chocolate can still have considerably higher carbs than what would be optimal for someone experiencing low tissue calcium problems like cramps. With this understanding, dark chocolate should be viewed as a better choice when it comes to treats than, say, a jelly doughnut. But it should not be viewed as something that is benefiting your health, as if you should have it everyday. That is just fiction that somebody made up to feel better about eating chocolate.

Now, let's all just calm down for a minute. Here comes the part where you let me be your friend again because I'm going to explain why you love that chocolate so much and what you can do to avoid your hopeless need for it. If you can correct your desperation for chocolate as well as for other carbs and sugars, you can drastically improve the level of cramps you are experiencing. The best part is that I don't think your cravings have anything to do with a lack of willpower, or that you're a "chocoholic," or anything like that. I know people have told you to just stop eating those things, but I'm here to tell you this: If you're having cravings, there is always an issue in your body chemistry that is creating those cravings. With many people, no amount of willpower is going to help them dodge their cravings. I will cover this more thoroughly when I release *Kick Cravings in the Nuts*, but I'll give you a quick overview here that could easily change your entire life. Seriously, this is huge.

Cravings - Part Two

I talked about cravings in chapter six, under *Electrolyte Deficiency Imbalance*. If you skipped that part, go back and read that now. I just want to review that topic so I can cover a few more aspects of cravings while I'm talking about carbs and sugars because this is a huge factor when it comes to cramps. "If sugar, chocolate and carbs are so bad for my cramps, why are my cravings around my period strong enough for me to consider holding up a 7-11?" That's an excellent question and I'm glad you asked. Like I said, you're about to get your hands on some life-changing information—cravings from the standpoint of your physiology.

Your blood pressure is a reflection of the salts (mineral content) in your system, as well as sugars and proteins a little bit, too. If your salts are low, you can have seizures. If your sugars are low, you can have seizures. If your salts and sugars are low at the same time, you have an even greater chance of experiencing seizures. If your *Imbalance Guide* showed indications of an Electrolyte Deficiency Imbalance, odds are pretty good that your mineral content is considerably low. This is usually why people crave salty foods, sweet and sugary foods, or carbs like bread or crackers (that can be converted to sugars). The body isn't so dumb. If salts are low, you can buffer them by raising your sugars and you'll be fine. The reverse is also true. If sugars are low, you can buffer them by raising your salts. The cravings are just your body's way of helping you to raise either your salts or your sugars in order to keep you from pushing toward seizures.

Remember, to get rid of cravings, people with low salts can raise their mineral content by:

1. Using unrefined salt (like sea salt).
2. Using specific supplements.
3. Correcting any digestion problems that are keeping the body from properly breaking down food, so the mineral content can be assimilated by the body. If you're not

digesting correctly, you're not getting the minerals out of your food.

If your urine pH is above 6.0, this factor may make your cravings even stronger. The higher your urine pH, the stronger your insulin can become. This is significant because if you eat sugars, starches or carbs and your insulin is stronger than normal, it can sweep too much sugar into your cells too quickly. This can push your blood sugar levels extremely low. If your mineral levels were already extremely low, and now your sugar levels are also too low, your body will literally begin to scream at you to do something about it. This "screaming" can show up in the form of intense thoughts about how nice it would be to eat some chocolate right now, or have a glass of wine, or some corn chips, or a cigarette, etc. Basically, anything that can constrict the vascular system or thicken up the blood and buffer either those low salts or sugars.

Are your cravings beginning to make sense now? Do you see that it really isn't your fault and the fact that you give in time and time again is just how the body was designed to continue functioning? Don't take what I'm writing here as permission to eat all this junk. That's not what I'm saying. The point I'm making is that there is a reason you have these cravings; and if you understand the science behind them, you can do something about them that is more ideal. Getting a grasp on the cause of your cravings is far more important than finding new ways to avoid giving in to them. Another way to look at it is this: Won't it be more fun to consume your chocolate from time to time as pure enjoyment, instead of needing it on a daily basis and feeling guilty every time you eat six cupcakes in a single sitting?

I talk about how to raise your mineral content and improve any digestive issues in chapter twelve. Is the suspense killing you? With how much I've been talking about chapter twelve I bet if I just left it out of the book completely, there would be riots in LA that would make you think the Lakers won another championship. (By the way, let me get this straight... your city wins a championship... so, you flip cars over and light them on fire. How do you explain yourself? I live in LA and just want to make sure my readers know that everyone that lives here is not that ignorant. I think Kobe has the ability to bring out the stupidity in some people.)

Chocolate seems to be the magic craving of choice. This may be due to its ability to both thicken and acidify the bloodstream. If an individual is pulling too much calcium out of the tissues and holding it in the bloodstream, that blood can lean too alkaline. When this happens, something called "The Bohr Effect" kicks in. The simple explanation is that when the blood is too alkaline, oxygen can't get down to the tissue level where it belongs. This can affect energy production and set up the terrain of those tissues for other types of malfunction. By eating something that can acidify the bloodstream, like chocolate, more oxygen can get down to the tissue level where it needs to be. In this regard, chocolate can not only thicken up the blood and raise your blood pressure, it can also help get more oxygen down to the tissues if your blood is leaning too alkaline.

If your *Imbalance Guide* shows that you may be leaning toward an Alkalosis issue, this could be contributing to your chocolate cravings. If chocolate is helping to lift your blood pressure and balance out the pH of your blood, your cravings would certainly be strong enough to talk you into downing enough chocolate to set yourself up for some nasty sugar-induced cramps. Improving any Electrolyte Deficiency Imbalance or Alkaline Imbalance could reduce the amount of chocolate you are craving.

L.A.'s Finest

I have a client who manages one of the most successful rock bands in the history of music. His son is also a client of mine. Obviously, this family is doing okay financially so they spare no expense when it comes to the health of their children. Before they

172

came to me, the son was having a lot of health issues so they sent him to this spiritual guru just outside of Hollywood. This guru was incredibly expensive and was recommended to them by some of their celebrity friends. The son (we'll call him Tommy, just like the kid who used to work on the docks) told me the story of visiting this guru and it might be one of my favorite stories of all time.

Tommy drove up into the mountains outside of Santa Monica to the address he was given for his "guru appointment." He parked in a small parking lot and followed the signs directing up a small, unpaved path. The winding path went up the side of mountain. He said it was exactly like what you would expect if you were climbing a mountain to see an old wise man. When he reached the top, he couldn't believe that an old wise man is exactly what he found. Inside of a small cabin on the top of a mountain, overlooking the ocean, sat a small bald man with a long gray beard. The guru asked Tommy to sit on a pillow on the floor in front of him. He told Tommy he was going to ask him a few questions about his troubles, and then they would sit in total silence for over an hour while he reached inside his aura to find the answers he was seeking.

The guru asked his questions and Tommy explained how he was having issues with headaches, nausea, and he couldn't sleep because his legs were always restless. The guru simply said, "I see." Tommy started to explain more, but the guru held up one finger signaling him not to speak and to close his eyes. For the next hour and half they sat in silence. Finally, the guru tapped Tommy on the forehead and Tommy knew he was about to receive an amazing piece of information. The guru looked him square in the eyes and said, "Don't eat sugar. That stuff's not good for you." That was it.

I told Tommy, "Man, this guy is a genius!" He puts on this whole show to get his point across, charges more money than O.J. Simpson's lawyer, and just tells people the one piece of information that could pretty much improve anyone's life: Don't eat sugar. This guy really is a guru.

Sugars And Complex Carbs

Now you get to learn the same piece of information that Tommy learned without paying a boatload of money or climbing to the top of a mountain. I know you love your sugar and your carbs, but at least you now have an understanding of why you love them. At least you now have the knowledge that when digestion is not working properly, the body likes these sugars and carbs because they are easier to digest and can be used to thicken up the blood in a person walking around with a low amount of minerals. Be sure to get the point that just because you understand why you like them doesn't make it okay to eat them all the time.

We learned from Dr. Melvin Page that it can take up to seventy-two hours for the body to recover from a carbohydrate event. What he meant by that was, every time we eat starches or higher amounts of carbohydrates, it creates a series of events that can take up to seventy-two hours for the body to regain its balance—almost as if eating those carbs creates all these jobs that the body has to deal with before it can recover.

In your scenario (a woman who wishes her cramps would leave her alone), this can be a tremendously big factor. In this book, I have outlined many steps you can take to improve menstrual cramps. However, if you're taking steps in the right direction, but huge leaps in the wrong direction, do you really think you're going to see great results? Next time you're in your car, try driving with your foot mashed down on the gas and the brake at the same time and see how good your results are. I recommend trying this as far away from people and telephone poles as possible. If you're going to put in the effort to improve your cramps, don't also continue doing the things that are likely creating them in the first place. If you know that sugar and carbs are going to pull calcium out of the tissues, and you know that low tissue calcium is one of the leading factors behind bad cramps, find a way out of that game.

My suggestion is to do the work to correct any digestive issues, do the work to bring more mineral into the system, and do the work to push more calcium down to the tissue level where it belongs. Once you start to see improvement, then, and only then, start trying to re-introduce some of the things you have cut back on. You may find that you can handle some chocolate or sugar on occasion once you have put your body in a healthier state. Yes, the chocolate or sugar is still going to pull calcium out of your tissues, because we know calcium will follow sugar and that's just how science works. In this scenario, however, you have increased the level of calcium currently in your tissues, so when some is pulled out, it does not leave behind such an incredible deficiency.

Whatever you do, don't just try to quit eating carbs and sugars like you're some kind of ninja. Be certain that you take the steps to improve any cravings you have, like I talked about in chapter six. If you don't straighten this out first, it's very unlikely that you'll be able to reduce your carbs or sugars without becoming a "less than pleasant" person. Especially if an Electrolyte Deficiency Imbalance showed up on your *Imbalance Guide*.

What Carbs Should I Eat?

Since you don't want to eliminate all your carbs if you have a low mineral content, it will help you to understand what carbs are the best to eat. The glycemic index explains the speed at which different carbohydrates convert to glucose and spike blood sugar. Searching for "Glycemic Index" on the Internet will bring up a variety of charts and tables showing the glycemic value of different foods. You might be surprised at some of the values you find. For example, potatoes have a glycemic value of 90 while white sugar is only 60. I'm not saying that white sugar should be a staple in your diet, but you can see that potatoes could be much more damaging to your cramps than some sugar could.

Another method to calculating optimal carb levels is to look at the "active carb" count of a food. Since fiber reduces how quickly the sugars or carbs in food hits your blood stream, the higher the fiber and the lower the carbs, the better. To figure out the active carbs just subtract the fiber from the carbs and that will give you the active carbs. (In other words, the carbs that will spike your insulin.) If you can keep those around 12-25 for as many meals as possible, you'll be doing yourself a big favor in the realm of reducing how much calcium you are pulling out of your tissues.

The main thought to keep in mind is that if you eliminate all carbs while your mineral content is low, you're going to have some crazy cravings, end up binging like a mad man, experience depression issues, or even worse, have a seizure. Your goal should be to include carbs that won't spike your blood sugar so high. Once you correct digestion issues and get more minerals in the system, you can reduce carbs further, if needed. You just don't want to drop your carbs too low in the beginning. Including higher fiber carbs that have a lower active carb count or are lower on the glycemic index is a great way to hold off your cravings for things like chocolate, sweets, and complex carbs like bread, potatoes, rice or pasta.

Hypoglycemics And Low Blood Sugar

Though reducing carbs and sugars is often crucial to improve cramps, about ten percent of the women who read this book will not be able to cut out carbohydrates and sugar, and still act like a reasonable human being. I skimmed over the fact that a higher urine pH can have the ability to make insulin too strong. This can contribute to blood sugar dropping too low. It is also common to see breath rate go higher than sixteen breaths a minute with these individuals. When blood sugar drops too low, any form of patience or rational thinking can go out the window. If you, or a loved one ever experiences this, you know exactly what I'm talking about. For these people, very low amounts of sugar may be necessary from time to time to keep their blood sugar from dropping too low. The way to really figure this out is to carry a glucometer with you. If you find that someone steps in front of you in the bank line, and you come close to jamming your pen into this person's ear, that would be a great time to check your blood sugar. If your glucometer reads below 70, you know it might be time for a small amount of sugar. Maybe in the form of some berries, or part of an apple, or some type of snack that contains sugar in small amounts. This is where a protein bar sweetened with xylitol or stevia could help.

Doing the work to perhaps lower your urine pH into a more balanced range could reduce this issue over the long haul, but if sugar levels are dropping too low, be sure to monitor your numbers, measure blood sugar, and take the necessary steps.

Mining Your Own Body

The machine that we call a human body needs resources to function correctly. Resources in the form of vitamins, minerals, amino acids, fats, etc., are needed to allow the body to complete the functions it handles from day to day, or even minute to minute. If digestion is not working properly, and food is not being fully broken down into these primary elements of nutrition, the needed resources are not coming in to the system. Fortunately, the body comes equipped with backup plan on top of backup plan when things don't go the way they should. These backup plans can sometimes cause trouble over the long-term; but when you think about it, some of these long-term problems are better choices than the body just not functioning at all by next week.

There is one specific backup plan that can greatly contribute to menstrual cramps. When your body is not getting the resources it needs from the food coming in, it still needs those resources and it will usually just go and find them. This is a problem because the 24-hour supermarket that your body is shopping from is YOU. Your body will mine the minerals and nutrients that it is looking

177

for from your own tissues and bones. Your body will literally break down your body in order to give your body the resources your body needs to operate your body (I just wanted to see how many times I could say "your body" in one sentence).

While the body is mining for nutrients, calcium tends to be among the minerals that are stripped from the tissues and bones. We already know that cramps are going to become more severe with a lack of calcium at the tissue level (tissue level means inside your cells). But what happens to our bones if calcium is stripped from them as well? Ever heard of osteoporosis? The medical world describes osteoporosis as if the body is "attacking" its own bones. This is a nice story for those who enjoy a good Braveheart-like epic tale, but doesn't it make more sense that the bones would become weak due to the fact that the body has no choice other than to break down this bone and use those minerals to keep the body functioning? I will cover this more in the upcoming *Kick Osteoporosis in the Nuts*, but this brief description is an excellent way to help you understand how the body will stop at nothing to get the resources it needs. Therefore, if digestion is not working properly, digestion becomes a top priority if your goal is to improve menstrual cramps. Otherwise, if the body can't get what it needs through digestion, it's going to continue looking elsewhere... and elsewhere is in your tissues and bones.

Resilience Of The Body

When I talk about resilience of the body, I'm describing the body's willingness and ability to return to the ideal state once presented with stresses from the environment. These stresses can originate from within the body, but they can also emanate from external sources. Think of it as your body's ability to adapt to its environment and the current circumstances. When you lose your resilience, you are in essence losing your health. Do you find that you are overly sensitive to some things? If you can't stand the atmospheric pressure, if you can't stand the heat, if you can't stand the cold, if you can't stand the sunlight, if chemical smells are hard to deal with—you're losing your ability to adapt to the environment. I have also heard people refer to this as adaptive capacity.

When looking at individuality, increasing people's resilience can do a lot for their well-being and how they move through life. However, I don't really view resilience as something to work on. Improving imbalances, digestive issues, and the other things I cover in this book will often allow the resilience of the body to become stronger naturally. I include this here because it's an excellent way to better understand how the body works. Understanding the resilience of the body and its importance can give you insight as to why the body might do something like pull minerals out of the tissues, even if this can cause a tissue mineral deficiency and result in more cramps. The body has great backup plans when it loses its ability to adapt to environmental factors. The part that sucks is that some of these backup plans can result in symptoms that are not so fun.

The anabolic/catabolic paradigm requires resilience to oscillate from one state to the other. In the morning, a person begins to transition from the anabolic (sleep time) state to a catabolic state, continuing in that direction until the late afternoon or evening hours. In these evening hours, the resilience of a person starts to push him back toward the anabolic state, because now the environmental tide of life, approaching the sunset of the day, signals the body to begin its push in this anabolic direction. This swing from anabolic to catabolic, and back to anabolic again, can be thought of much like a pendulum.

The problem is, some individuals have very little resilience in their system. Stated another way, they have very little "reserve energy." The result is that their pendulum begins to have less and less swing. This helps us understand one variable that could allow people to get stuck in one state or the other. If there isn't enough "umph" to make a switch from the anabolic state to the catabolic state, or vice-versa, these people just might live most of their lives in the state they are stuck in. Another possibility is they may switch states every two weeks or so instead of twice a day, depending on how low their reserve energy is.

When I'm picking a piece of fruit to eat, like an apple or a peach, it's nice if that fruit is not too hard. On the other hand, it is easy for fruit to become very mushy. I don't want mushy fruit anymore than I want a mushy handshake. Shake my hand, dammit. Whether looking at the hard fruit or the mushy fruit, either side indicates that there is not the proper resilience to show that the fruit is in an ideal state of being ready for consumption. Trees are meant to bend in the wind, and it's their resilience that lets them go back to their original shape; deadwood breaks off in the wind because it has no resilience.

When a person climbs the stairs, blood pressure will normally increase to accept the "load" of climbing the stairs. Resilience allows for blood pressure to return to its proper state when the person is no longer stressed by climbing the stairs. If the blood pressure stays up all the time, this person is unable to return to an ideal state.

Are you starting to get the idea? Most of the time, trouble that shows up in the human body stems from no longer having the ability to adapt to environmental factors—a loss of resilience.

Stress

People always say stress is bad for you but they never say why. Anger, stress, frustration and all those emotions seen as danger (thereby justifying a need for energy) can cause the body to lift sugar levels that metabolize to create acids and hormonal chemicals in your body. All these chemicals are just more garbage your body has to deal with. It's like eating a Ding Dong. When you eat processed junk food, your body has to deal with those chemicals and sugars. The chemicals created from your stress have to be dealt with by the body too. Your body can only do so much at once. If it is dealing with chemicals from stress at a time that it could have been removing some toxin that was brought in from a food or pollutant, now these other toxins can end up being stored as fat since the body is busy elsewhere. That's what the body does with a lot of junk that it can't deal with at the time. It just shoves it into fat cells to make the toxin inert and harmless to the body. In this regard, can stress make you fat? In a roundabout way, I guess it can.

Under stress, your body will also take blood and energy away from the digestive processes to deal with the immediate threat (the threat being whatever is causing you stress). Your body doesn't know that you're stressed merely because you're stuck in traffic. To your body, your interpretation of stress is equal to, "We're being chased by a lion so create chemicals that will help us get away from a lion." Under stress, your body will also push more glucose into the bloodstream to be used as immediate energy. When glucose levels go high, insulin has to go high to handle that glucose. When insulin levels go high, the body can't burn stored fat for fuel and it will even send the signal to pack away *more* fat. Look at that, stress is making you fat again. For crying out loud, calm down!

I don't know how stressed you actually are. If it's a lot, start thinking about ways that you can process these stressful situations in your life in a more calming manner. Or see if you can find a little time for yourself to relax in some way, even if it's just stopping and taking a deep breath a few times a day. I know this is more work, but keep it in your mind and start to investigate things that you might enjoy that can reduce the stress in your life because *your* stress is a huge stress on *your* body. The body is already under a lot of stress. Not only is it stressed to remove toxins and pollutants, or fight off invaders that have set up a college party town in your body, stress can also be induced by a lack of resources. I've talked a lot in this book about different circumstances that can result in a lack of resources within the body. Well, a lack of resources is a stress to the body. "How am I going to pay $800 worth of bills with $15?" That's the type of situation your body has to figure out when it needs a large number of resources and there aren't enough coming in due to a lack of digestion or poor diet choices.

Diet choices! There's another possible stress to the body. Do you really think your body was made to consume squirt cheese? This is not food. This is not what your body was made to run on. The things we call food these days are enough to stress out any human body. Let's say you worked on an assembly line and your job was to pick up the square pegs off the conveyor belt and place them in the boxes. One day, instead of square pegs on the conveyor belt, you started seeing balloon animals. Your supervisor is nowhere to be seen. You know that if you get behind again you're going to be fired, so you just have to do the best you can at cramming the inflated poodle balloons into boxes that were made for square pegs. This would be stressful. This is what many of our bodies go through every day. The body has to figure out this scramble of, "How do I take this substance that was not made for consumption and process it with a digestive system that was made to process real food?" Help your body out and eat something that comes from the earth instead of a package in a vending machine.

Sun Exposure

It's important to remember that when your body is exposed to the sun, it creates its own vitamin D. This means that sun exposure is like taking vitamin D. That doesn't mean that you can't go into the sun. But if your cramps are bad, and you can see that your tissue calcium is likely low, you might want to stay out of the sun until you get your cramps under control. If you do go into the sun, be sure to take some type of fatty acid or L-Lysine to help push the calcium back into the tissues. The idea is to try to reverse what the vitamin D is going to do, which is pull calcium out of the tissues.

Sea Salt

Most people never use salt because we're always taught that it's not healthy. And that can be true... for some people. For people who have high blood pressure because their bodies don't have the ability to wash out junk, then sometimes adding salt for those people may only raise their blood pressure further. But for people who have a low mineral content and low blood pressure, a quality sea salt can literally change their life. Sea salt is, in essence, minerals from the sea. It also contains a chloride ion that is necessary for your body to make its own HCL. Without this chloride ion, people can't make enough HCL to properly digest their food.

Some people tell me that they don't like salt. Usually this is because they have associated decreased health with using salt so they begin to avoid it. However, as your body realizes, "Hey, we can really use this stuff for a lot of functions," your taste buds will change, you will begin to really like the taste and you'll even crave it. Just be sure to get a good brand. I really like a brand called Celtic Sea Salt. They have one variety that is really big chunks and is harder to use, but they also have a few fine versions which pour just like table salt; I like those. But this is important: Their normal fine version is okay but it doesn't have enough mineral to really help individuals who showed a strong Electrolyte Deficiency Imbalance on their *Imbalance Guide.* The one that can be like a wonder drug for people who are severely electrolyte deficient is called "Flower of the Ocean" by Celtic Sea Salt. It's very expensive so look at it like buying a supplement and not like buying salt. If you can't find Celtic Sea Salt, most Himalayan sea salts are also good in a pinch, in my opinion. If you think I was making an idiotic pun-like joke with the "pinch" in reference to salt, I will be furious.

Bonus Insight

This one is free of charge. It has been my experience that many electrolyte deficient people who are also catabolic seem to instinctively gravitate away from eating salt. They learn that if they stop eating salt they will not have diarrhea because the decrease in salt intake will inhibit HCL production. In chapter eight, I mentioned that too much HCL production could cause diarrhea for some people with poor bile flow. These details are found under *Crohns, Colitis, & IBS* if you would like to go back and review. In any case, if the individuals I'm talking about can improve their bile flow, they can often go back to using salt without any problems.

CHAPTER TEN

Foods That Can Help

The search for a diet that works for everyone can stop now. Really. Shut it down. It's not gonna happen. You're better off wasting your time looking for a chocolate fountain of youth. Wasn't it Ponce De Leon himself who once said, "This diet is pissing me off and I have yet to lose a single pound." Look at it realistically—if one diet worked for everybody, why are there so many diets?

As soon as you adopt a new base understanding that there is no diet that is right for every person, and there is no supplement that is right for every person, then you can stop throwing your time in the garbage looking for the magic diet or the "silver bullet." There are foods and supplements that can bring about changes in your body that will make you feel as if they have a magical effect, but they won't bring about the same results for your sister or even your neighbor who grows her fingernails way too long to not be considered creepy. Since they don't work for everyone, they're really not magic are they? They are just the more ideal choice for you and your chemistry. With this new understanding, you can now switch your attention from finding the quick fix "superfood" and move your energy toward using foods and supplements that are more advantageous for your specific body and its needs.

I really like the idea of using food choices to improve imbalances. Hippocrates said, "Let your food be your medicine and your medicine be your food." Seeing how Hippocrates is considered to be the "father of western medicine," I'm pretty sure western medicine stopped listening to Daddy at some point. It seems you would have a real hard time finding a medical doctor who would give you any advice about food at all. It's true some doctors are given a poster of a food pyramid and you can even look at it on the wall while your doctor fills out your prescriptions. I have clients with Type II Diabetes who tell me that their doctors never mentioned food to them. Even with Type II Diabetes our doctors don't seem to be teaching their patients that sugars and starches have the ability to quickly raise blood sugar levels that are already too high, as levels often are in diabetics. (By the way, I love that the Hippocratic oath is to "do no harm." Do you really want someone working on you who's trying to "do no harm?" How about someone who's trying to do some good?)

Food (or non-food in many cases) is what fuels our bodies. If you don't think the type of fuel you eat matters, try putting anything in the gas tank of your car other than what was intended to go there: gas. If you really don't believe me, fill your car's gas tank with Gatorade or soda or Oreo cookies and then drive back to the bookstore so you can return this book. If you make it to the store, you're right. If not, you can read the rest of this book while you wait for AAA to pick you up. Just don't get upset if the tow truck driver wants to take a picture of you so he can show all his friends the person who crammed cookies into the gas tank. We really are smarter than this as a civilization. When we think about it, it's obvious. It's just very hard for us to see this concept when we have been taught only one way our whole lives. At least we now have the ability to open our eyes, if only a little.

Below I list food choices that can affect specific imbalances. For each imbalance, I list foods that seem to commonly improve that imbalance and other foods that appear to most frequently push a person further into that imbalance. Keep in mind that you are still

186

an individual and foods that commonly push an imbalance one direction for most people may have an opposite reaction with you. That is why it is so important for you to monitor what you're doing and how your chemistry is moving. Because different individuals have different digestive predispositions and capacities, the same food can have a different effect on similar imbalances from person to person.

It's a lot of fun finding specific foods that can make you feel better, but most people cannot count on food alone. In nearly every case of a severe imbalance, those people's chemistries have been moving further out of balance for years or even decades. They have likely been making less than ideal choices for a long, long time. To push that chemistry back into balance, it's reasonable to think that they would have to make the right food choices for just as long, if their goal was to become balanced. That is not a scientific formula so don't hold too much weight in what I just said. It's just a good analogy so calm down and don't try to pull out a calendar to figure out the exact day in your life when you began to eat poorly. The point I'm trying to get across is that sometimes it will take more than food alone to straighten out a severe imbalance. But in most cases, eating foods that benefit an imbalance can reduce the required effort in other areas (like supplementation) so that you can reach your goals faster.

Supplements are a much more concentrated form of specific nutrients than what can be found in most foods. Some supplements are even made of what are called "complete foods" or "whole foods." No, not from the store, Whole Foods. These phrases just mean that these supplements are made from food instead of from a synthetic, fractionated form of that nutrient. I talk more about these supplements in chapter eleven. I like to see people use supplements along with the correct food choices in order to see results faster, and then gradually reduce the amount of supplements they need until they can keep their body balanced with food choices alone. With that goal in mind, I spend this chapter digging into the foods that can be beneficial for each imbalance.

My final warning about this chapter goes like this: If you have a severe imbalance that may be contributing to your cramps, and you see a food listed under an "avoid" column for that imbalance, that doesn't mean you can never eat that food again. You can eat that food tomorrow if you want—you'll just be slowing down your results. For example, soft-boiled eggs normally have the ability to push a person more anabolic. If you have a severe Anabolic Imbalance, the best plan is to avoid soft-boiled eggs until you become more balanced. But maybe you have a requirement in your life that makes it impossible to avoid soft-boiled eggs. Maybe you are part of a very specific religion that prays only to chickens and you feel that cooking the egg too much will bring a thunderstorm that would wipe out your crops... or something like that. (I'm pretty sure I'm not supposed to make fun of different religions but I'm going to go ahead and take my chances making fun of the "chanting to chickens, leaving the egg yolk runny" religion.) If you are a card-carrying member of the "chicken people" and still need to eat soft-boiled eggs, you can try to increase your anti-anabolic protocol in other areas to allow you to eat a food that is going to push you the wrong direction (more anabolic). Maybe you need to really increase your food intake that will push you less anabolic. Maybe you can add another supplement to make up for it.

It is optimal to avoid the foods that will make a severe imbalance worse, but you do have some options. You can get creative if you feel as though removing a food is not an option for you. You will learn that even the time of day that a food or supplement is implemented matters. This may allow you to keep some of your favorite foods in the mix by simply adjusting what time of the day you eat them.

Diet Is Determined By Strength Of Digestion

Instead of selecting your diet from the last magazine article you read, you might want to try eating according to what your digestion can handle. Yes, the goal is to correct digestive issues so you can broaden your selection. However, while you're doing the work to improve digestion, try adjusting your food selection according to your ability to digest.

If your HCL production appears to be low, proteins may be harder to digest. If your bile is not flowing properly, fats can be difficult to emulsify and process. If you've become insulin resistant, you can have a hard time correctly processing carbohydrates and you may want to reduce the amount of starches you are eating. Understanding your current situation can help you better gauge what type of foods you should avoid and what foods you should eat.

This is more proof that there is no diet that is right for every person. Let's learn to help individuals based on each person's individual needs, not based on categories of people.

Contradictions From Imbalance To Imbalance

You may notice that if you are dealing with more than one imbalance, "foods to implement" and "foods to avoid" may contradict each other from imbalance to imbalance. For example, foods that are recommended to help an Anabolic Imbalance may also be recommended to avoid for an Electrolyte Deficiency Imbalance. If you come across a similar circumstance, you can try to avoid any foods that have the ability to push either imbalance further out of whack. Alternately, if you have one imbalance that is severe, and one that is only a slight imbalance, you can try to focus on the foods that will benefit the severe imbalance, even if those foods are not optimal for the slight imbalance that you are dealing with. You may need to see what works best for you by watching your self-test numbers when you eat these foods. Keep in mind that a higher priority imbalance will normally be favored over a lower priority imbalance, as discussed in chapter five.

Some of you are going to take the suggestions below and turn them into "rules" rather than suggestions based on principles. When a child is very young, you give him a lot of rules. "Stay in your yard." "Don't chase the ball into the street." "Don't read books which start with the title 'Kick It in the Nuts.'" As the child reaches the teen years, the parents have to settle with just saying, "Be careful." The parents have to hope the child has the sense to apply, to the current circumstance, the principles suggested by those previous rules. So please do not allow me to be more than a friend offering suggestions to think about.

You really only need to read about the foods below that are listed under the imbalances that showed up on your *Imbalance Guide*. I don't mind if you want to read about the foods that benefit each imbalance, just don't confuse yourself by soaking in information that does not apply to you and your chemistry. I am hoping that you've already performed your self-tests and know which imbalances you are dealing with so you can at least understand which imbalances to focus on the most. If you have not run your self-tests, is it because you hate me? Run your self-tests already.

Imbalance - Electrolyte Deficiency

Avoid

- Avoid not properly digesting your food.
  Many adults do not have their digestion functioning optimally and they have no idea that there is even a problem. Chapter seven smacked you in the face for many pages on this subject so I won't yell at you again about it, but if this imbalance showed up for you, DO NOT ignore digestion.
- Avoid drinking too much water or being unconscious about water intake.

This doesn't mean you don't need more water, you may. However, you need to qualify to drink more water. If you have a low amount of minerals in the system, drinking a lot of water will just wash away the small amount you do have. Work on correcting digestion and increasing your sea salt intake and then you can increase your water as your blood pressure comes up.

- Avoid drinking distilled water or tap water.
  Since distilled water contains no minerals, drinking it can wash minerals out without replenishing them. Chlorine and fluoride in tap water can also reduce minerals in the body since the body needs to use those minerals to help safely remove the chlorine and fluoride from the body.

- Avoid eating too many sugars and especially starchy carbohydrates.
  If you recall, your blood pressure is made up not only of mineral in the system, but also sugars (and some proteins too). If you overindulge in sugars or, especially, starches that convert to sugars, this overindulgence can trigger an insulin response that is too fast and strong which could clear too much sugar out of the system. If you're a person with low mineral levels, now your sugars are low and your minerals are low, leaving the body with very little to operate with. Keeping sugars and insulin levels on an even keel can be very beneficial for someone with an Electrolyte Deficiency Imbalance.

Implement

- Eating food.
  This means eating breakfast. Often because digestion is not functioning properly, understandably, many people skip breakfast. After all, why eat protein for breakfast when it's going to make you feel miserable for the next six hours? But if the mineral level is low because of poor digestion, as digestion is repaired, something needs to be given to the body to digest. Once the body sees that it has the ability to pull nutrients out of the food you're eating,

191

the body is going to want more of that. Remember, if digestion is functioning, digestion allows food to become your medicine. Diet is what you eat, nutrition is what your cells see after the food has been broken down to elemental parts.

- Tomatoes and/or tomato sauce.
Tomatoes have the ability to thicken your blood, thereby raising your blood pressure. If you like tomato sauce, using it is a great way to make just about any meal beneficial for an Electrolyte Deficiency Imbalance.

- Using an unrefined sea salt with your food.
In my opinion, when it comes to food, unrefined sea salt can be the most important component to implement for an Electrolyte Deficiency Imbalance. Yes, it is true that correcting any digestive issues takes center stage for this imbalance. However, if you're not getting enough chloride into your system, your body can't begin to make its own HCL in the stomach. This is often the missing factor when a person has digestive issues. In chapter eight, I explained how a lack of HCL is not the only issue that can keep digestion from working correctly—but it does seem to be the most frequent.

If this imbalance appeared to be severe on your Imbalance Guide, a good unrefined sea salt has the ability to create some amazing changes. But you may be an individual who needs to be aggressive with the salt. When I have clients with extremely low blood pressure and all the numbers are pointing to a severe Electrolyte Deficiency Imbalance, I like to see them load up the sea salt at every meal as much as they can. I tell them that if they are eating lunch with a friend, the goal should be to use so much salt that your friend cries out, "What the hell is wrong with you?"

Obviously, you don't want to make your food gross. Don't add so much salt that you can't get through your meal

192

without gagging. But if you can add salt to your meal, take a bite and it still tastes okay, you might want to add a little more. Just stop before it begins to taste like a salt lick. If you don't know what a salt lick is, google "salt lick" or "mineral lick." You will be intrigued by what you find. People use salt licks with horses a lot. It's kind of funny to see that many horse owners don't really understand why they give it to their horses. They just hear that it's beneficial so they do it. Nature photographers use a salt lick to attract wildlife. Animals will come from far and wide to load up on needed minerals. Yet, we humans still view salt as if it's a bad thing. Oops.

The word salary even comes from "salt." In Roman times, soldiers were paid in salt. Would you go to work every day and fight for your life if they were paying you in salt? Maybe you should. Maybe your life would be better since you would probably use some of that salt.

I'm not positive, but I believe it was Mother Theresa who once said, "Salt 'em if ya got 'em."

Imbalance - Electrolyte Excess

Avoid

- Avoid drinking tap water that is loaded with chlorine and/or fluoride.
  You may notice that I recommend avoiding some of the same things for opposite imbalances. For example, I've listed avoiding tap water under Electrolyte Deficiency as well as Electrolyte Excess. Logic might tell you that if an item is bad for one imbalance, it should be good for the opposite imbalance. However, that is not always the case. It can sometimes be beneficial to avoid a specific item from imbalance to imbalance, and for totally different reasons.

For an Electrolyte Deficiency Imbalance, it was recommended to avoid tap water containing chlorine or fluoride because drinking this water can strip the body of needed minerals. With an Electrolyte Excess Imbalance, tap water should also be avoided but for different reasons. If the body's waste removal systems are not working optimally, chemicals from the tap water can build up, making the bloodstream thicker and harder to keep clean. Remember, with an Electrolyte Excess Imbalance, the blood is often too thick so it doesn't help to bring in more filth and muddy up the system. Drinking adequate water is fundamental in helping the kidneys. In this regard, intake of clean water can equate to changing the bag in the vacuum cleaners of the blood.

- Avoid eating too many sugars or starchy carbohydrates.
  Sugars and carbohydrates can thicken the blood; therefore, excessive consumption is not recommended with an Electrolyte Excess Imbalance. Measuring blood sugar with a glucometer can be helpful.

- Avoid taking antacids.
  Antacids restrict proper digestion, as discussed in chapter eight. Undigested foods become a waste product that the body has to deal with. Normally with an Electrolyte Excess Imbalance, the body is already having trouble removing excess junk or mineral from the system. Therefore, antacids that turn most of your food into undigested junk may place a heavier burden on your body.

- Avoid eating polyunsaturated oils (such as salad dressings, margarine, mayonnaise and foods fried or cooked with vegetable oils). Coconut oil, real butter and unheated virgin olive oil are all okay.

Implement

- Using an unrefined sea salt with your food.
  The initial thought for someone with an Electrolyte Excess Imbalance would be to avoid salt. It is true that if you add

194

salt with this imbalance, you will want to monitor your blood pressure and make sure it does not go up. However, if adding sea salt can provide the body with the chloride needed to improve HCL production, higher HCL production can improve digestion, therefore reducing the junk in the system that was created as a result of improper digestion. Now, the body has one less burden and can focus on removing waste. This can help the body reduce blood pressure.

- Correcting any digestive issues so you can properly break down your food.
- Drinking more water.
- Eating a lot of low-starch green vegetables.

Imbalance - Anabolic

Avoid
- Avoid foods made with hydrogenated and polyunsaturated fatty acids: canola, corn and soy oils
- Avoid ice cream
- Avoid butter
- Avoid cream
- Avoid cheese
- Avoid juices
- Avoid foods made with sugar
- Avoid coffee
- Avoid tea
- Avoid soda
- Avoid excessive fruit
- Avoid vinegar
- Avoid poached or soft-boiled eggs

Implement
- Non-starchy vegetables
- Fish (especially salmon)

- Unheated virgin olive oil
- Flax seed oil (in a pearl-type gelcap is best; do not heat flax seed oil)
- Ground flax seed
- Lemon juice
- Citrus fruit
- Sardines
- Tuna fish
- Fried or omelet-style eggs in the morning (not Egg-Beaters or egg whites).

    Even in a time crunch, if you make hard-boiled eggs, you can keep them in the fridge and grab one on the run in the morning. When your digestion is working correctly, a hard-boiled or hard-cooked egg can be a powerful anti-anabolic meal and can even reduce your need for anti-anabolic supplements.

Powerful Anti-Anabolic Meal

There is a widely used recipe from the Budwig Diet that I feel to be very anti-anabolic inducing. It's basically cottage cheese and flax seed oil blended together with ground flax seed stirred in, but there are specifics that you have to follow for the science to work.

The reasons this recipe works are: First, it contains all the fatty acids to help push a person less anabolic, and second, when the sulfur proteins in the cottage cheese are blended at the molecular level with the fatty acids, a sulfur compound that can get into the cells where needed is created. Sulfur is a very strong anti-anabolic substance.

This is the recipe:
1. Take 3 Tbs of extra virgin olive oil. (The Budwig Diet calls for cold-pressed flax seed oil, but it appears that most flax seed oil sold in stores is rancid before it leaves the shelves. Freshly made flax seed oil would be acceptable, but it can

196

be hard to find. The extra virgin olive oil is an excellent replacement.)

2. Blend with 6 Tbs of cottage cheese. Stirring them together will not work. They need to be blended so that the molecules join together. An immersion blender is the best way to do that because one serving is too small to put in a blender or food processor. One of those hand held, single blade immersion blenders is best, but a juice blender will do too. Blend the first two ingredients for about a minute. It will look like pudding.

3. Grind 2 Tbs of fresh flax seeds (a coffee grinder works well and will probably cost you about $30). It's important to grind them fresh because the lignans will lose their effectiveness after about 30 minutes. For this reason, the ground flax seed from the store does not work the same. Once ground, just stir it into the cottage cheese mixture with a spoon.

4. Optional: Add broken up walnuts or Brazil nuts. Make sure they are raw and not roasted.

If you're super anabolic, eating this whenever you have time may be beneficial, but earlier in the day is more optimal than at night since people are meant to be more catabolic during the day. Therefore, this dish is best eaten at breakfast or as a snack before lunch.

Imbalance - Catabolic

Avoid

- Avoid flax seed oil
- Avoid fish oils
- Avoid DHEA
- Avoid fried foods
- Avoid canned or processed meats and fish
- Avoid foods made with hydrogenated and polyunsaturated fatty acids: canola, corn and soy oils

- If you eat fried or hard-boiled eggs, eat them only in the morning and limit them

Implement
- Poached or soft-boiled eggs, especially at night
- Non-starchy vegetables
- Real butter/cream
- Fresh cheeses such as cottage, mozzarella, and cream cheese (these are not aged cheeses)
- Coconut oil

Coconut Yummies

Coconut oil can be beneficial in a variety of ways. One, it contains saturated fats which are pro-anabolic. Two, it can dramatically aid in weight loss by giving you the healthy fats your body needs in order for it to willingly let go of stored fats. Three, coconut oil stands up to heat better than other common kitchen oils, which makes it the best choice to cook with. At first, coconut oil may taste a little different with some foods, like eggs. However, sooner or later your body will realize it can really utilize coconut oil, your taste buds will change, and you will end up enjoying it much more than any other oil. All that being said, cooking with it alone is usually not enough to get crazy weight loss or pro-anabolic results.

My favorite trick is to melt a cup of coconut oil in the oven or a toaster oven. You can also melt your coconut oil by placing the container in hot water in the sink. Either method can take a few minutes, but do not use a microwave just because it may be quicker! Next, I stir in half a packet of stevia and about 20-40 drops of flavored stevia. Optionally, you can open up four or five capsules of Pau D' Arco and mix them in too. Pau D' Arco is an herb commonly used for its anti-microbial properties, but it can add an almost chocolate-like taste to the coconut oil. As an alternative, you can add cinnamon or mint if you prefer those flavors.

To mold the coconut oil into little treats, I use silicone mini-muffin baking dishes. You can see the type I use under BOOK TOOLS > HELPFUL LINKS at www.KickItInTheNuts.com
I put about a tablespoon or tablespoon and a half in each mini-muffin hole and put the batch in the fridge to harden.

These Coconut Yummies make a nice after-meal mint that also helps me burn fat and may push my chemistry more anabolic. Or, if you're more advanced and you think the coconut oil tastes good enough to simply eat a teaspoon of it plain with a meal, that will work too. I'm just fancy.

In the summer, you will notice that coconut oil often turns liquid because it melts at room temperature; it will usually stay solid in the winter.

Just be sure to eat coconut oil either with a meal or right after a meal because you want that digestive activity going on from your food to help emulsify the fats in the coconut oil so they can be properly utilized. Try to consume between a teaspoon and a tablespoon of coconut oil near meals two or three times a day when you're home. It is unlikely that you're going to pull coconut oil out of your pocket at a restaurant; but when you're home, it's easy to use.

Imbalance - Tricarb Fast Oxidizer (Carb Burner)

Avoid

- Avoid sugar and similar items like corn syrup and honey.
- Avoid fruit juices and large quantities of fruit.
- Avoid coffee, tea, and alcohol.
- Avoid eating polyunsaturated oils (such as salad dressings, margarine, mayonnaise and foods fried or cooked with vegetable oils). Coconut oil, real butter, and unheated virgin olive oil are okay.

- Avoid meals consisting predominantly of sugars or starches. It could be beneficial for you to include at least a small serving of protein and healthy fats in each meal.

Implement

- Non-starch vegetables that can provide carbs without such a high level of carbs that the meal spikes your insulin levels. Vegetables like zucchini, squash, broccoli and asparagus can be beneficial.
- Eating some carbs early in the day, but try to avoid meals made up predominantly of carbs.
- Keep your glucometer on you at all times. Knowing when your blood sugar is low will allow you to manage your blood sugar instead of being at the mercy of it.

Imbalance - Beta Slow Oxidizer (Fat Burner)

While you are improving this imbalance, it is important to reduce your starch and sugar intake. (Keep in mind that if you experience drops in your blood sugar and you need starches or sugars from time to time in order to continue functioning, small amounts of sugar will often bring a better result than starches will. But for most people with this imbalance, limiting intake of both starches and sugars will be beneficial.) When you reduce one type of nutrient, another type must be increased to fill in the gaps. I like to increase fat intake with this imbalance since the body appears to be burning fat well. However, it is important that bile is flowing properly so you can emulsify those fats. If you increase fat intake, and bile is not flowing well, it could result in weight gain or breakouts caused by the body trying to push fats that have not been emulsified out of the body through the skin. Read about digestive supplements in chapter twelve to see if you need to work on your bile flow before increasing your fat intake.

Avoid

- Avoid sugar and similar items like corn syrup and honey.

- Avoid fruit juices and large quantities of fruit.
- Avoid drinking alcohol and soda.
- Avoid eating polyunsaturated oils (such as salad dressings, margarine, mayonnaise and foods fried or cooked with vegetable oils). Coconut oil, real butter, and unheated virgin olive oil are okay.
- Avoid meals consisting predominantly of sugars or starches. It could be beneficial for you to include at least a small serving of protein and healthy fats in each meal.

Implement
- Consuming good fats like coconut oil, real butter, unheated virgin olive oil, and those found in eggs (the whole egg) or animal proteins.
- Keep your glucometer on you for measuring when your blood sugar is high or low. This will allow you to manage blood sugar instead of being at the mercy of it.

Imbalance - Parasympathetic

Avoid
- Avoid starch, and limit sugar and similar items like corn syrup and honey. (If you experience drops in blood sugar, small amounts of sugar can help you to continue avoiding starches.)
- Avoid fruit juices and large quantities of fruit.
- Avoid eating polyunsaturated oils (such as salad dressings, margarine, mayonnaise and foods fried or cooked with vegetable oils). Coconut oil, real butter, and unheated virgin olive oil are okay.
- Avoid meals consisting predominantly of sugars or starches. It could be beneficial for you to include at least a small serving of protein and healthy fats in each meal.

Implement

- Any supplements needed to improve digestion if digestive issues are present. (See chapter twelve.)

Imbalance - Sympathetic

Avoid

- Avoid starch, and limit sugar and similar items like corn syrup and honey. (If you experience drops in blood sugar, small amounts of sugar can help you to continue avoiding starches.)
- Avoid xanthines like coffee, tea, chocolate, and cola.
- Avoid any soda containing phosphoric acid.
- Avoid canned and processed meats.
- Avoid eating polyunsaturated oils (such as salad dressings, margarine, mayonnaise and foods fried or cooked with vegetable oils). Coconut oil, real butter, and unheated virgin olive oil are okay.

Implement

- Relaxation techniques and eating in a relaxed state.

Imbalance - Tending To Acidosis

When looking at an Acid Imbalance, it's very important that you don't use the popular view of "alkalizing" to improve this issue. There are lists all over the internet of foods that are said to be alkalizing; yet not only are the views on these lists inappropriate, I find those lists to be very misleading.

These food lists often refer to "alkaline ash" or "acid ash" food items. The method used to make this designation is this: A food such as a lemon is burned up and then its ash is mixed with water. If the pH of that ash comes up alkaline, the ash residue defines that the food is to be regarded as an alkaline-inducing food. First of all, there is nothing in digestion that resembles a fire. If a very exquisite building burned to the ground, would people pick up the ash of that building and say that the ash is "exquisite building inducing"? No, they wouldn't. The ash no longer has form. Function follows form. Since the building's form was destroyed in fire, the ash no longer functions in any way close to the building. In this same way, the aqueous chemistry of the food that was burnt up cannot become a predictor of how the fresh food behaves. How would you feel in a restaurant if you asked for some lemon in your water and they sprinkled some ash from burnt lemons into your glass? Do you think it would taste the same as a fresh lemon?

First of all, remember that an Acid Imbalance is referring to your blood pH and this may not necessarily be reflected by your urine pH or saliva pH. Most of those "alkalizing food" lists are telling us that if we eat those foods, we will watch our urine pH and saliva pH come up. That is not our goal in improving an Acid Imbalance. With an Acid Imbalance, we would like to see our breath rate go down and our breath hold time get longer. Second, it's my experience that most of those lists are not very true. Remember, for any food to have any type of an effect on you, it first needs to be properly broken down by your digestive system; and there is a large percentage of the population that does not have their digestion working very well. That's why I always tell people that if they don't have their digestion working well, it really doesn't matter what they eat because it's all just going to either rot and ferment in the system, or move too quickly through the system to be properly assimilated by the body. With that in mind, if you want to move urine pH or saliva pH one direction or the other, the best advice I can give you is to register on *The Coalition* and use the pH balancing chart tool so you can see where your current numbers are and what foods and supplements can push you the right direction. To improve an Acid Imbalance, however, here are some things I have seen create good results.

Avoid
- Avoid fruit juices and large quantities of fruit.

- Avoid eating polyunsaturated oils (such as salad dressings, margarine, mayonnaise and foods fried or cooked with vegetable oils). Coconut oil, real butter, and unheated virgin olive oil are okay.
- Avoid soda (plain soda water is okay).

Implement

- Eating more green vegetables.
- Drinking more water.
- Choline is a nutrient that can be very helpful in alkalizing one's bloodstream and egg yolks contain a high amount of choline. In this respect, egg yolks could be a beneficial food for an Acid Imbalance.

Imbalance - Tending To Alkalosis

Avoid

- Avoid drinking too much "alkalizing" water. (I talked a little about people making an effort to "alkalize their body" in chapter six, so if you weren't paying attention, go back and read that again. This can be important if you have an Alkaline Imbalance or compromised stomach HCL production.)
- Avoid using any form of "alkalizing supplements."
- Avoid using antacids.
- Avoid eating too many sugars and starches. (If you experience drops in blood sugar, small amounts of sugar can help you to continue avoiding starches.)

Implement

- Using unrefined sea salt with your food.
- Eating protein. (Not bigger servings of protein, but more frequent servings of poultry, eggs, fish, or meat.)

CHAPTER ELEVEN

Using Supplements

It seems we are always hearing something good or bad about supplements in the news or in health magazines. The truth is, the media is all correct in some way or another—all the good and all the bad. Since every person is different and is experiencing different imbalances, specific supplements can either correct that person's imbalance or exacerbate it. Beyond the fact that we really need to use the right supplements that will benefit our biological individuality, we also need to use supplements that the body can assimilate. Many supplements on the market today are not worth the bottle they're sold in. I'll teach you what to look for and where to get quality supplements that are right for you. Since many readers will need the aid of supplements in order to improve their cramps, don't take this information lightly. You don't want to waste your money on supplements that are not effective for you.

Many supplements that you can buy in the store are junk. What's worse is it appears that they may even be made that way intentionally. Most vitamins, minerals and herbs have the ability to move body chemistry. The problem is that most consumers don't know anything about body chemistry and what vitamins will move that chemistry which direction. Wouldn't it make sense that if the vitamin manufacturers didn't want to deal with lawsuits all day long, they could just add binders to the supplements that make them very hard to assimilate?

Binders, lubricants and fillers are often added to supplements to hold tablets together, improve the ability for the supplements to run through the processing machinery faster and easier, or to make the supplements cheaper to manufacture. Any number of these added ingredients can reduce your body's ability to assimilate the nutrients found in those supplements. It is said that, with most consumer-based supplements, you can assimilate only between 4-12% of what's in them. In that way, it's difficult for people to push their chemistry the wrong way and there's no lawsuit. Whether companies are adding these binders to save money or to avoid lawsuits really doesn't matter. Either way, you still don't get an effective product.

There are companies that make high quality supplements without the harmful binders in them. The trick is most of these companies sell their products only to qualified health care practitioners. In that way, if there's a lawsuit, it falls on the practitioner and not on the company.

That's why you always hear so much good and bad about supplements. They are only good if you use the good ones, and they're only good if you know what should be used with your specific body chemistry. Most people choose a supplement because they read that it is good for a specific symptom. Little do they understand that a chemical imbalance is normally causing that symptom. If the supplement they choose can help correct that imbalance, they may see good results. If it doesn't, they will see bad results. Remember, one symptom can have many different underlying causes, so it is very common that two different people with the same symptom can experience very different results using the same supplement. Have I mentioned that it's not a good idea to treat your symptoms? If you don't wake up at least once in the middle of the night hearing me say, "Don't treat your symptoms," I will have failed in my efforts to teach you to look at your underlying causes measured using chemistry instead of looking at your symptoms. Since you now have a better idea of where your chemistry is, you have an edge that most people never get to experience. Welcome to where all the cool kids hang out.

A lot of issues can be corrected with food choices alone. I mentioned in chapter ten that if a person has been pushing an imbalance the wrong way for a decade, it could take eating all the right foods for another decade to push it back. For this reason, I spend plenty of time in chapters twelve and thirteen going over supplements that can help correct each imbalance faster than some food choices could. Once an imbalance is corrected, most people can often stay on track with proper food choices and they no longer need to use most of the supplements unless they see their chemistry moving back in the wrong direction. For example, beets and beet greens are excellent foods that will help your bile flow better. But instead of eating a bucket of beet tops every day, many people use a whole/complete food concentrated form of beets and beet greens called Beet Flow. It's a more convenient way to get in a bucket of beet tops every day.

Understand this: You're not going to be able to pop a few supplements and correct everything that's been going wrong for the past fifteen years. Supplements are not witchcraft. You're going to have to find a way to eliminate some of the things that are making these imbalances worse and add in new choices that will help you correct them. Any supplement usage is just a boost to help it happen quicker. None of the supplements I talk about in this book are intended to be used indefinitely like an over-the-counter drug often can be. These supplements are meant to correct deficiency or excess issues, and then a person should reduce what they're using until they don't need them anymore. Enzymes are the only exception; I explain that in chapter twelve when I go over digestive supplements. Frequently, when people start to work on their bodies, they may need to use a lot of supplements in the beginning to get things going in the right direction, but they will be able to reduce supplements as imbalances get corrected.

What If I Hate Taking Supplements?

No problem. You always have the option to continue being miserable (yes, I understand I'm a jackass). The truth is, many people will be able to greatly improve their situation with food choices alone, or maybe just adding a good sea salt. I see that happen all the time. I also see people who are so screwed up, not only do they really need the help of good supplements, they often need the help of a lot of them in the beginning.

Once you get in the habit of using supplements, it can be as easy as washing your hair. Yet, it's very interesting how averse some people are to using supplements at all. I have talked with people who have been suffering for years or even decades from issues like insomnia, constipation or diarrhea. They tell me that they don't like to put anything unknown in their body. That's okay. I can understand wanting to keep bad stuff out of your body. But with chronic issues like those mentioned, your body is screaming at you that things are not going as planned and it could really use some help. Take the time to learn more about supplements that could help you so you can feel good about using them.

I've already gone over why we hear so many good and bad stories about supplements. Yet, if you know which supplements are appropriate for you, and how to find the good ones, you're miles ahead of most people. Beyond all that, don't you think it's a little silly to avoid supplements because you're not sure what they're going to do to your body, yet you feel great about keeping candy bars in your desk that contain chemicals and artificial sweeteners that you *know* are harmful? It's up to you to make your own decisions. All I can do is point out how ridiculous some of your decisions are.

Don't view taking a lot of supplements as popping a bunch of pills. Most natural supplements are concentrated forms of specific nutrients, many made directly from food itself. So, you can view these supplements as part of your food. It's a much more convenient way to get the specific nutrients your body is looking for, rather than needing to shop at fifteen different farmer's markets to find a specific type of beet green. Who has time for that? If you view the supplements as the bane of your existence, you're obviously not going to feel good about taking them and they are clearly not going to be able to bring their full benefit. However, if you view them as a convenient way to cheat and reach your goals faster, they can make your life a whole lot easier.

I can't recommend specific supplements to you so don't waste your time emailing me questions about what you should be using. There are legal ramifications that don't allow me to help in that regard. But in this book, I can show you which supplements appear to help correct certain imbalances and I can even tell you what supplements I may take if I were trying to correct an imbalance. After you have that information you can decide for yourself if you want to try anything.

Where To Find It

If I'm going to buy supplements from a store, I try to avoid the large, national chain supplement stores. This is not a rule, but it is my experience that the bigger the national chain supplement store, the more garbage they sell in that store. As a way to recognize natural products as being the best in their field, my company, www.ShapeYou.com, developed a program called the GearAwards. I find that most of the manufacturers that sell products in these big national supplement stores can't even meet the requirements to submit their products to our awards program, much less have a chance of winning anything. Generally speaking, we allow only natural product submissions. Most products on the market today contain too many chemicals, binders and just plain junk to even be considered. Again, this is not a rule. There are certainly large companies out there doing the right thing.

While many companies are doing something right, very few companies are doing everything correctly. I try to sort through more than one factor when trying to decide which companies really deserve a gold star. But most of the products from these large companies that are doing the right thing can also be found in health food stores and independently owned supplement shops. These are the places where I buy my products if I'm going to buy from a store.

Buying products online can be a good idea too. When I do buy online, I try to find the most natural product. If a product has twenty ingredients listed under "Other Ingredients," and you can't pronounce most of them, that's probably not a very clean product. By clean I mean it's not filled with a bunch of junk that your body doesn't need and likely won't know what to do with.

What To Look For

Most supplements list the contents on the nutrition label. They state the nutrients that are in each capsule, the serving size, the amount in each serving, and sometimes even the percentage of the suggested daily allowance that the serving will provide. You often see this as "%DV." For example, if the label lists fifteen percent for calcium, it means one serving provides fifteen percent of the minimum amount you need each day, according to what government studies suggest. If you think that I believe all of those percentages are crap, you would be correct. If you've read this far, you know each person is different.

Below the nutrition facts you normally see "Other Ingredients." This is where you can see what type of garbage the manufacturers are really putting in their products. If the other ingredients include "Gelatin (capsule), rice bran," that's a pretty clean supplement. It's hard to beat that unless they use only a gelatin capsule and nothing else. (This happens to be my favorite scenario but is often hard to find because so many products are difficult to run through the machines without something that makes the encapsulation process easier and keeps the machines from getting gummed up.) Let's look at a few key words to keep an eye out for and what they might mean for you.

Di-Calcium Phosphate

You will see this product listed under "Other Ingredients" in just about every cheaply made supplement out there. This is the cheapest substance that makes the manufacturing process the easiest. The problem is di-calcium phosphate actually restricts your body's ability to absorb nutrients—not only the nutrients in the supplement that you're taking, but also any other nutrients that you consume. So, not only is it likely that you're not getting the benefits from the supplement that you are taking, you are likely also reducing the benefits of any food that you eat with it. Does that mean I would continue to use this supplement? Yes, I would use it to fill my garbage and I would never buy it again. When someone asks my opinion on a product that contains di-calcium phosphate, my response is always, "Who told you to take this? Do they hate you?"

Magnesium Stearate

There is a lot of argument out there about magnesium stearate as well. Some feel the way magnesium stearate is processed can cause it to contain harmful additives, while others feel that magnesium stearate contains beneficial factors. I try to avoid it when I can. But some products are just too hard to encapsulate without it so it's pretty common to see. Both sides of this argument are intriguing, but I have yet to see conclusive evidence like I have for di-calcium phosphate. So, when I can avoid magnesium stearate, I do. But I don't junk an entire product if it contains some in the "Other Ingredients."

Gelatin vs. Vegetable Capsules

First of all, I really do prefer to see a capsule over a tablet, as capsules are generally easier to dissolve and assimilate. However, there are a few whole food/complete food supplement companies out there that make excellent tablets and I will talk about them next. As far as capsule preference goes, gelatin is by far a superior product. If you are vegan and not willing to use animal products in your supplements, a vegetable capsule can be okay. But generally speaking, vegetable capsules are much harder to break down than gelatin.

Since I already mentioned that some people need help with supplementation in order to get their digestion working correctly, how are they going to correct their digestion if they can't even dissolve the capsule that is supposed to help them digest? Since I like supplements to work, I prefer a gelatin capsule. But if you have beliefs, like chickens and cows have the right to live freely among us, then I support your choices and advocate the use of vegetable capsules as well. But if you're a person who is just as happy kicking a cat as you are petting it, then go with the gelatin capsule because you will get a better result. (Before you send your letters, I have never kicked a cat nor any other animal and I am quite the animal lover, but yes, I did laugh when I wrote that.)

Whole Food/Complete Food Supplements

Whole food/complete food supplements means that these supplements are made from just that, whole foods. It's like putting actual food into supplement form. The goal is to include the entire spectrum of the nutrient, just as you would find it in food, so the body can use it as nature intended. I am a fan of this type of manufacturing and I often use many whole food supplements.

Since I talk about vitamin C next, I'll use that as an example. Many varieties of "vitamin C" that are sold in stores today are just a synthetic fraction of the vitamin C structure. Ascorbic acid is a form of vitamin C, and it does have many beneficial uses—but it is not the complete C vitamin. In order to properly use ascorbic acid as vitamin C, the body has to pull all the necessary co-factors out

212

of the body's reserves in order to form a complete vitamin C. With these additions, the body can use the nutrient for good. The problem is, after several days, the body will run out of the cofactors that are being pulled from your reserves to make the ascorbic acid a complete C. Then you're ingesting just a fraction of the vitamin C that cannot be used for the different types of repair processes in the body.

In order to get the full benefit from vitamin C, you need to take a whole food/complete food form of vitamin C—one that contains all the needed cofactors so that the vitamin can be used properly. Standard Process and Empirical Labs are well respected whole food supplement manufacturers. Standard Process sells their products only through health care professionals. In order to purchase these products, you would need to find a practitioner who is qualified to order Standard Process supplements. At www.NaturalReference.com you will find a variety of Empirical Labs products, some of which are available to consumers and some that are sold only to health care professionals. Many products from Empirical Labs are specifically designed to move the imbalances I have been talking about in this book, and those products must be purchased through a qualified health coach. Empirical Labs has a whole food vitamin C called Bio-C that I like a lot.

Professional health coaches use a variety of supplements from different companies in order to help their clients move chemistry to a more balanced state. In this book, I mention only companies and supplements that I am familiar with. That doesn't mean the supplements I mention are the only options. Quality, contents, and "other ingredients" in each product vary too greatly for me to be able to talk intelligently about products I know nothing about.

Please don't think that just because a supplement is made from complete food that it is a good supplement. If the food is not dense with nutrients, that kind of misses the point, don't you think? In this regard, the manufacturer still needs to be using foods that were farmed in a manner that allows nutrients to exist at high levels in those foods. I talk more about nutrient density in chapter fourteen. For now, avoid viewing a whole food/complete food supplement as perfect. The supplement still needs to be manufactured well.

To add a word of warning, be careful where you buy your quality supplement brands if you're buying them online. There is a trend going on where dishonest people slap a well-known company label on a bottle of sugar pills and sell it as something else. It's not very hard to Photoshop a label and print it off. I mention www.NaturalReference.com a lot because I know they are a certified retailer for a lot of the supplements I mention in this book. If you buy supplements elsewhere, it can be a good idea to call the manufacturer and make sure the site you are buying from is a legitimate seller of that brand.

Vitamin C

Vitamin C is used in nearly every type of repair process that the body performs. The body can also use vitamin C to attach to harmful toxins so those toxins can be safely removed from the body. We also use vitamin C to re-reduce glutathione and make it potent in its ability to stop free-radical activity. So, we really use vitamin C a lot. The problem is that humans, primates and guinea pigs are the only mammals that don't make their own vitamin C. We have to get it from our diet. But in this country, there's not a sufficient amount in our diet.

Some symptoms of a vitamin C deficiency can be:
- coated tongue
- bruise easily
- frequent colds
- slow to heal
- pink toothbrush (bleeding gums)

Ascorbic acid (like I talked about above under *Whole Food/Complete Food Supplements*) and other fractions of the C vitamin can still be very helpful in adding weight to the correct side of an imbalance. Nonetheless, to improve a vitamin C deficiency, one would need to use a supplement like Bio-C (or similar product) that gathers more of the co-factors that your body requires to use the vitamin C.

I find that most people can benefit from some type of whole food vitamin C. If you used the 11-parameter dipsticks in your self-assessment, there is a measurement for vitamin C on that dipstick that will indicate if you have sufficient vitamin C to the point that your body is willing to excrete some in the urine. If you are C deficient, it's a great idea to start using enough vitamin C every day until that deficiency doesn't show up on the dipstick anymore, and then maintain a good level by using that supplement a few times a week. If you are vitamin C deficient, it could be because you're not getting enough in your diet. Or maybe you are getting enough in your diet but your body is just dealing with something that is causing the vitamin C to be used up faster than you can bring it in. Either way, a whole food vitamin C could be very beneficial.

Check with a health coach to see if vitamin C supplementation is right for you. On the 11-parameter dipstick, a reading that shows plenty of ascorbic acid (a form of vitamin C) being peed out could indicate that you are getting plenty of C. However, adequate vitamin C coming out in your urine can also be a result of being in an overly catabolic and disintegrating state. This is when the assistance of a professional health coach could help you discern whether or not to continue any vitamin C supplementation.

When To Take Supplements

The time of day you take specific supplements can make a big difference. Next, I list the optimal times that each type of nutrient should be taken. Just understand that I'm talking about only the

215

optimal times. For most supplements, if you take them with your meal or right before your meal, it's going to be okay. There will always be exceptions to this rule and there will be supplements that need to be taken away from meals. My point is that life is short; don't make yourself miserable trying to take your supplements at exactly the time that I outline below if that is something that is hard to fit into your life. If you can get in what you need, in most cases that will be beneficial to you and that's really what you're looking for. The main goal is to have a convenient way to increase the good nutrients you're taking in. Beyond the guidelines below, some digestive supplements have very specific times to be taken and I cover those in chapter twelve.

Vitamins

Most vitamins, like C or B vitamins, can be taken with or away from a meal because they will be absorbed into the system either way.

Minerals

Minerals are easier to assimilate when aided by the act of digestion and should therefore be taken with a meal, when possible. There are liquid mineral supplements I use that seem to be easy to assimilate whether they are taken with a meal or without. But when it comes to minerals in capsules or tablets, taking them with a meal is a good rule to try to follow since some minerals in certain forms are harder to absorb than others.

Amino Acids

Amino acids can be absorbed into the system with or without food, just like vitamins. However, the optimal time to take amino acids is between meals. Thirty minutes before a meal is best, but that can be hard to remember and fit into your day. If you can do it, great; but if this is too inconvenient and it's just going to make you forget to take them, then I suggest taking them with your meal.

L-Glutamine is an exception to this rule when it comes to amino acids. I like to see L-Glutamine taken away from protein because L-Glutamine will compete with protein for absorption. Therefore, taking it with protein will reduce your ability to assimilate both the L-Glutamine and the protein that you're eating in that meal.

Single amino acids have the ability to correct problems and also induce problems if not used carefully. For this reason, more than casual attention needs to be given to monitoring your numbers and checking if they have moved to a range that would allow you to reduce the use of any specific amino acid.

Digestive Enzymes

It is best to take these with meals. Digestive enzymes should be used indefinitely anytime cooked or processed foods are consumed. I discuss digestive enzymes further in chapter twelve.

Probiotics

Probiotics have been getting a lot more mainstream attention lately. Scores of people are realizing the benefits of probiotic use. Interesting. Does this mean the medical world might eventually have to admit that it is the overuse of their antibiotics that is creating the problems that the probiotics are helping? I do believe that some of the probiotic talk is going a little overboard in the way that many people are telling us to use them all the time. The truth is, if the terrain is right in the gut, good bacteria will colonize—if it's not, they won't. It's kind of like grass. If the terrain is right, the grass is going to grow. You can even find a blade of grass in a little crack in the sidewalk in the middle of New York City. If the terrain is right in that crack, grass will grow.

Probiotics are an excellent tool and should be used to recolonize the beneficial bacteria in your gut, but indefinite use is required only if you have diarrhea. Because anytime you have diarrhea, you've fried 'em. I also like the idea of using more than one type of probiotic to introduce a wider variety of beneficial bacteria strands. Using probiotics for a couple weeks is often plenty. It's best to take most probiotics away from food. Just before bed or right when you wake up are great times. And beware of probiotic products that are sugar-fied to the level of being Kool-Aid.

CHAPTER TWELVE

Digestive Supplements

Well, here we are... the long awaited chapter twelve! Boy, this chapter better have some kind of fairy dust in it or I will have built it up way too much. In all actuality, I have seen people use some of the guidelines found in this chapter and feel like they did come across some type of magical potion. But that is not the case. The body can do some amazing things on its own once it begins bringing in the nutrients it needs through proper digestion.

For this particular book, most readers could probably use some type of digestive help. Even if digestive issues didn't show up on your *Imbalance Guide*, but an Electrolyte Deficiency Imbalance did, I would still look to boost your digestion until your Electrolyte Deficiency Imbalance has improved. If you're missing periods or your cramps are severe, I would also look to improve digestion until those issues have improved. If you have digestive issues that you don't address through using supplements, foods or supplements used to correct other imbalances may not have the effect you are hoping for. Digestion needs to be working correctly in order for most other supplements to be effective. Don't take this lightly. If you're not using digestive enzymes, I would at least look to add those into your routine since they are a key factor in proper digestion. Not everyone needs to improve digestion, but anyone over the age of thirty should probably be using digestive enzymes.

There is no digestive supplement I recommend to everyone unless I'm just talking about enzymes. I still want to look at what the person's specific needs are. Do you recall how I talked about the way digestion works? The quick review is that acid is created in the stomach; then, that acid mixed with the food you ate moves into the duodenum where the bile drops on it and creates a sizzle that breaks food into elemental nutrients. It's that sizzle we're really looking for. You need both the acid production and the bile flow to get that sizzle. Other things like pancreatic enzymes and bicarb will function automatically in most cases if you have that bile dropping. Your main concerns are the acid production and the bile flow. I get to digestive enzymes later, but acid production and bile flow are the priorities that I'll go over first.

Hydrochloric Acid (HCL) Warning

Hydrochloric Acid (HCL), also known as Betaine HCL, is the most widely needed digestive supplement in my opinion. It's also the one that comes with the most important instructions. This is NOT a supplement you want to take willy-nilly. (Isn't it amazing that such a ridiculous phrase like "willy-nilly" could become so widely accepted? That bugs me.) If you're going to be using HCL, I recommend coming back and reviewing the next section every week for the first few weeks, just to make sure you're doing everything correctly. That way, you won't be willy or nilly.

Also, if you're going to use HCL, be sure to also use Beet Flow, or a similar product. I never allow any of my clients to use HCL unless they are also using Beet Flow. If you don't' have your bile flowing correctly, and you add more acid into the stomach, you could create a duodenal ulcer or diarrhea issues. I cover Beet Flow and bile in more detail later in this chapter. I just want to make sure you understand not to use HCL without also using Beet Flow.

HCL Protocol

Judicious use of HCL supplementation starts breaking down your food to release and ionize the minerals from the food. Your body starts to assimilate those minerals, adding to your mineral reserves, and the HCL production starts to naturally increase again. While you do this, the minerals you are now getting from the food will also help to balance your body.

The goal should be to use a specific dose of HCL capsules, as described below, until you start to feel a warming in your stomach fifteen to twenty minutes after you eat; or you no longer experience any burping, bloating, digestive discomfort. You also want to make sure you are no longer seeing any undigested food in your stool. Though, you will need to pay attention to what you're doing, and it is possible to create loose stool issues or other discomforts if HCL is used incorrectly, many of you will not be able to fully restore digestion without using HCL.

In the middle of a meal with protein, take one HCL capsule. (It is important to chase HCL with at least one bite of food. If the capsule were to get stuck in your esophagus and dissolve there, it would feel a lot like heartburn.) The amount of HCL used is also measured against the amount of protein in the meal—more protein, more HCL; less protein, less HCL. If you do not feel a warming sensation in your tummy after that meal, take two HCL capsules at the next meal. If you do not then feel a warming sensation in your tummy, take three at the next meal. This process continues until you feel a warming sensation in your stomach, up to a maximum of five 500 mg capsules. Hold at this dosage until you feel a warming sensation in your tummy. Once this happens, at the next meal, back off one capsule and stay at that dosage for all successive meals until you begin to feel a warming sensation again, then back off another capsule and stay at that dosage level for successive meals. When you begin to feel a warming sensation again, back off another capsule. Continue to do this until you are down to one HCL capsule with each meal. When you feel a warming sensation after taking the single capsule, stop taking HCL supplements as your body now appears to be producing enough HCL on its own. Keep in mind, whatever your normal dosage is (say you are currently at five HCL), if you eat a meal with far less protein than you normally consume, you

221

may need only two or three HCL capsules with that meal, since it contains less protein. Many of you, will perhaps have no problem holding at five HCL per meal no matter what the protein level is for a given meal. Adjustment according to protein level is normally more important once your stomach is making more of its own acid. Then you may approach the level when you need to back down by one capsule.

What If I Don't Feel A Warming Sensation?

You may need to hold at the five HCL dosage for some time before your body can begin producing more HCL on its own. This process can take months for some individuals. The good news is that, even if your body is having trouble creating enough of its own HCL, you're still bringing it into the body through supplementation. Therefore, you are still improving your digestion. If you're not feeling a warming sensation after meals with five HCL, it's likely that your body may not have the mineral resources to make its own HCL. You can continue to take the five HCL dose until you eventually feel the warming in your stomach.

It is my experience that some individuals never feel a warming sensation. That's okay. You can also judge when it's time to reduce your dose of HCL by whether or not you are burping or bloating. The burping can just be small burps so don't think you need to belch one out to be considered a person who is burping. Small burps count too. Are you bloating? If you feel like your clothes fit tighter in the evening when you take them off than when you put them on, you're bloating. In either of these cases, perhaps your body is not making enough of its own HCL to warrant a reduction in your dose. However, if you stop burping and bloating, it may be time to try reducing your HCL dose by one capsule, as described previously in this chapter. Later in this chapter, I talk about other factors, like H. pylori, that can delay your body's ability to make its own HCL. Even feeling anxious while you're eating can inhibit HCL production. If you're eating with someone you don't like, make sure you take your HCL

222

capsules so they don't blow your digestion and affect the rest of your day.

What If I Take Too Much?

The dose of your HCL should be judged against how much protein is in each meal. You may have to play with this a little bit to figure out what is best for you. The higher the level of protein in that meal, the more HCL you need. The dose is still going to be in the same range of what you have found to work for you. Just because you enter an all-you-can-eat ribs contest doesn't mean that you need to take 30 HCL capsules. You might simply adjust your normal dose by two or three, depending on the protein content. For example, a salad with only vegetables would require far less HCL than a meal consisting of a chicken breast or a ribeye steak and steamed broccoli. Make sense? If you misjudge the size of a meal and take too many HCL capsules, resulting in an upset stomach from too much acid, you can mix 1/4 - 1/2 teaspoon of baking soda in water and drink it. The baking soda will neutralize the acid. You will have eliminated proper digestion for that meal, but it may be a better option than the discomfort of having too much acid in your stomach. Then, at your next meal of the same protein content, adjust your HCL intake accordingly.

Ox bile products could also be used in a circumstance of taking too much HCL. Of course, using ox bile right after a meal will still stop digestion similar to baking soda. I talk more about ox bile products later in this chapter, but Empirical Labs makes an ox bile product called Bil-E-Mulsion that I like for this purpose.

What If My Stool Becomes Too Loose?

If you begin to use HCL supplements and your stool becomes very loose and/or you experience extreme urgency to use the restroom (number two style), you may now have more acid coming from the stomach than your bile can cool off and neutralize. The body moves this acid product through the intestines quickly so as to not burn the intestinal lining. This doesn't necessarily mean that you don't have a need for that additional HCL; it may just mean that you don't have the proper bile flow to cool it off.

To use an illustration, let's say that your stomach's HCL production was at a 3 out of 5 (so you would need additional HCL supplementation to fully break down your food), but your bile flow was only at a 1 out of 5. That low amount of bile flow may not be enough to neutralize that acid and your stool could become loose. It may even come shooting out the back door like those flames that came out of the race car's tailpipe in *Grease*. You might need to temporarily reduce your HCL supplementation until you can correct the issues that are restricting your bile flow (I talk about how to work on that issue in just a minute). Once bile flow is correctly restored, you may be able to increase your HCL supplementation until you feel the warming in your tummy without experiencing any loose stool issues. Be sure to read the section *HCL With A Catabolic Imbalance* if you experience this "flaming ass" type situation.

What If I Feel Heartburn?

Like I talked about in chapter eight, marketing for this common complaint may be more misleading than just about any other health issue, but heartburn and reflux medications are literally a billion dollar industry on their own—so it's understandable. There are a few different causes of reflux; but very few, if any, are actually caused by too much acid as they explain when marketing their products. If you've learned anything in this book thus far, it's that every symptom can have multiple causes. To learn more about reflux, check out *Kick Reflux, Heartburn, & GERD in the Nuts*, once it is released, because I focus on only one possible cause here.

In order to make this point, I'm going to review some topics from chapter eight:

- At the bottom of the esophagus is the LES, or lower esophageal sphincter. This valve opens to let food enter the stomach and then closes so that digested food doesn't go back up the esophagus and burn you. Sometimes people have a small hiatal hernia where part of the stomach is pulled up above the diaphragm keeping that valve from closing, and this can cause reflux for some sufferers.

- The most common cause of reflux: The LES is actually HCL sensitive, meaning that when the stomach makes enough HCL, it activates that valve to close so digesting food doesn't reflux back up. The problem is, a body that doesn't have all the mineral it needs can't produce enough HCL in the stomach to trigger the valve; reflux is the result. People aren't having reflux because of too much acid; they're having reflux because there is not enough acid.

- Pharmaceutical companies sell us drugs that turn the acid off, so that when we experience reflux, we can't feel the burning and we assume the originating issue has been dealt with. The problem with that is twofold:

  1. The stomach also contains digestive enzymes that can come back up with reflux. These digestive enzymes are made to break down protein. What is the esophagus made of? Yes, protein. Therefore, using these drugs stops the burning sensation, but it doesn't stop the damage that reflux can cause.

  2. These drugs stop digestion. There's a reason your stomach makes acid, but the medical community still tells you it's a good idea to turn that off. I already discussed this in detail in chapter eight. I simply want to remind you here that bile is one half of the critical digestive process, but the acid is

the other half; you must have both parts working correctly to properly digest the food you eat.

"But I never had reflux before, why am I having it now that I'm supplementing HCL?" I hear this question a lot. If you feel heartburn when you start to use HCL, and that is something new for you, that's just an indication that you didn't have enough stomach acid to feel that reflux. If you stay on track and continue to increase the HCL, that heartburn should reduce or go away completely by the time you reach a full dose of five 500 mg capsules. Below, I talk about one more factor that can contribute to this heartburn; but if you follow the guidelines I lay out in this book, and you still don't see any relief from your newly found heartburn, read *Kick Reflux, Heartburn, & GERD in the Nuts*, when available, because there may be other more complicated issues that you may have silently been dealing with for some time.

Eating Carbs When You First Start Using HCL

Here comes the classic mistake that can pop up when someone tries to use HCL supplementation for the first time. What feeds bacteria? Starch, sugar and carbohydrates. So, the person thinks, "I am going to take this HCL and I think I'll start with two pills." Depending on the content of the brand she is using, she would likely be taking somewhere around 1000 milligrams of hydrochloric acid; and this is really going to enhance her digestion. This is a good thing to do. Except, if we were to look inside her stomach we probably would find it's almost white with bacteria growth (since she had no acid before to kill all this bacteria).

To continue the story, this girl takes her 1000mg of hydrochloric acid and then she eats pancakes. Well, that is not going to be sufficient hydrochloric acid on her first dose to totally retard and negate that bacterial activity in the stomach. Now that she augmented her stomach acid (what little bit her body is producing along with 1000mg of hydrochloric acid from the two capsules), when this stuff comes up her esophagus because she still has a garden of bacteria growing, it is going to burn her like she's never been burned before. Once those pancakes come in, that bacteria gets all happy and jazzy and begins to create more gases. These gases are what cause the food to push back up her esophagus. As I said above, this is just one possible cause for acid reflux; but this seems to be pretty common for people who *really* need HCL and are just beginning to use supplementation.

When I say, "someone really needs HCL," I mean that individual has very little stomach acid. When there is very little stomach acid being produced, it's almost a guarantee that the person has some type of bacteria growth in the stomach. Bacteria is everywhere. Without that acid defense barrier that kills all the bad guys as they are coming in the castle, it just seems that bacteria have found a way to get in there and set up camp. Once this person gets up to a dose of HCL that is high enough to restrict the bacteria's activity, or high enough to trigger the LES valve to close, the reflux will greatly improve or stop altogether. Many forms of bacteria will die once your stomach acid is high enough; but a common bacteria, H. pylori, can be a little bastard and a little harder to kill. I'll include more about H. pylori in a minute if you just hold your horses. (My Mom used to say that to me a lot and I never had the heart to tell her that her favorite sayings don't make much sense.)

In my example above, the two HCL capsules were not enough to trigger the LES to close and the carbs consumed caused the bacteria to create more gasses so the reflux was severe. The low dose of HCL in the beginning is still a necessary step because people can't just start taking five HCL capsules in their first dose. If your body is making some HCL on its own, and you add in a stockpile more, the result will be way too much acid and that could be a very uncomfortable situation. This is why it is so important to start with just one capsule and work your way up each meal. By removing high carbohydrate foods (like bread, rice, pasta, cereal, sugar, etc.), you won't feed the bacteria that create those extra gasses and make any reflux more severe. It's just a good idea to play it safe and leave out the carbs while you're working up to your full dose of HCL. If it's hard for you to eliminate carbs at breakfast, for example, and it can be easier for you to remove carbs at lunch and dinner, just use the HCL capsules with lunch and dinner. Once you're up to the full dose of HCL, you can try to use them with carbs as well, since the HCL level should be high enough to trigger the LES to close.

H. Pylori

Time to cover H. Pylori in more depth now. In the world of research, it is commonly assumed that the decline in HCL production observed through later adult life (approximately 30% of the population over 65 years old doesn't make enough HCL) is a "normal" and common consequence of getting older. However, recent studies have indicated that the secretion of HCL does not decrease in the stomach as a person ages; HCL production actually appears to increase, especially in men. Even more evidence shows that the frequently observed reduction or loss of HCL production is generally the result of asymptomatic infections. The most common infection of this type for humans is Helicobacter pylori, or I'll just say H. pylori like all the fancy people say.

It is now a popular opinion that the older you are, the better your chances that you currently have an H. pylori infection. That percentage even goes up with each year of life that you have under your belt. For example, a 40-year-old person would have a 40% chance of having an H. pylori infection. I'm not a fan of treating according to the "at your age you need..." point of view, but these numbers do give a good indication of how common an H. pylori infection can be.

The chances of an H. pylori infection goes up drastically if you have ever used any type of acid reflux or heartburn medication that turns off stomach acid. Many believe that it is difficult for H.

pylori to colonize in a stomach with sufficient stomach acid; but if that level of stomach acid is temporarily reduced, H. pylori can invade and then find ways to survive once the production of stomach acid returns. It appears that H. pylori have the ability to crawl up into the mucous lining of the stomach, escape the acid during digestion, and then come back out once acid levels have dropped again. I believe that is why, if people with an H. pylori infection begin to use HCL supplementation or other products designed to kill H. pylori, those people will experience some improvement in their reflux symptoms. Yet, they won't experience complete eradication unless they take extra measures.

H. pylori can be such a major factor with digestion because this bacteria eats hydrogen. Hydrogen is what your body uses to mix with chloride to make HCL. If H. pylori is eating all of your hydrogen, your body won't be able to make very much HCL. I discussed earlier how countless people who are not making enough stomach acid likely don't have the minerals needed to make HCL. But you can see how an H. pylori infection could scarf up enough hydrogen to remove the other important factor in HCL production: The hydrogen.

Most of the acid reflux and heartburn medications out there are proton pump inhibitors, or PPIs, as they are called. They work by turning off the proton pump that makes hydrogen. Now the body can't make HCL anymore, so the person doesn't feel the reflux and the symptom is gone, just like I talked about earlier. But these drugs were actually developed to take care of H. pylori. By turning off hydrogen, you can starve H. pylori and they die. It just turned out that scientists realized turning off HCL production (and therefore digestion) could remove the symptoms of any reflux or heartburn, so they began marketing PPI products in that manner.

The compelling detail about these PPI drugs is that they can starve H. pylori, yet your odds of having an H. pylori infection increase if you've ever used one of these drugs. How could that be? Since you asked, I guess I'll tell you. It is widely accepted that most people won't start making hydrogen again for up to three weeks after they have ceased taking any type of proton pump inhibitor medication. This means people are not making HCL as long as they can't make hydrogen. Consequently, even if the lack of hydrogen starves the H. pylori out of existence, the acid-free "window of opportunity" is open for two or three weeks for any little bastards to come in and set up camp. You may recall I talked about how H. pylori can exist in an acid stomach as long as they get in while the acid levels are low. Isn't it realistic that H. pylori could make their way back in while people are barely starting to make hydrogen again? Maybe individuals are making enough hydrogen to feed bacteria, but not enough to create the acid barrier that keeps them all out.

This lack of acid barrier can also allow other types of bacteria in the front door—other bacteria that may live on sugar instead of hydrogen. If these bacteria can flourish in the three-week window of an acid-free environment in the stomach, they can create an alkaline environment that could stay more alkaline even after the body begins making HCL again. The waste product from most bacteria is alkaline, therefore making the environment more inhabitable for them. Do you see how just having the door open can set up the environment for H. pylori to re-infect the body? This isn't even considering the fact that, once you turn some people's digestion off, they have a hard time getting it started again. Seeing that the body can't break down what is being eaten well enough to pull the minerals out of the food, that individual may not have enough minerals needed for the body to make HCL again once the hydrogen turns back on. This shows how easy it can be for people to lose their optimal digestion for weeks, months, or even years. No matter how you chalk it up, you can see the wide variety of circumstances that could allow a bacterial infection to make its way into the body.

You may recall how reflux, or heartburn, is often caused by the activity of bacteria in the stomach. Doctors who deal with this issue a lot often tell me that, when they test for an infection in the stomach, they almost always find H. pylori and maybe some other type of pathogen as well. When symptoms of a bacterial infection in the stomach are present, H. pylori is very commonly at least one of the culprits. Other than creating common digestive symptoms like reflux, heartburn, or decreased ability to digest food, an H. pylori infection could exist for years, or even decades, without showing any real symptoms. Therefore, this infection will very often go undiagnosed. The new DNA stool tests that your doctor can order can be expensive if your insurance doesn't cover them; but it can be nice to know if you have an infection or not. Even without lab tests to confirm the presence of H. pylori, I've seen people just use supplemental products as if they have an infection since most products used to fight H. pylori would be acceptable for temporary use whether you had an infection or not.

Before you become too aggressive towards an H. pylori infection you are not certain exists, it might be best to take steps to improve digestion first. Since you may be dealing with a number of imbalances at first, the extra supplements it can take to wipe out an H. pylori infection could be overwhelming. I like to see someone first add HCL supplementation; additional HCL is usually all that is needed to increase acid production. If HCL capsules do not correct the problem and you feel like you may be dealing with H. pylori infection, using the information described below may be the best bet for you. You could also enlist the help of a professional health coach, as they may be able to better understand some of your numbers and determine if an H. pylori test, or supplement protocol is right for you.

Side note: If a person is dealing with a Sympathetic Imbalance, (maybe they are constantly stressed or living at the speed of light) this stress can also restrict a person's ability to properly produce sufficient HCL. If this sounds familiar, an excellent option may be to simply calm down before you jump to the conclusion that you must have an H. pylori infection.

I will go into H. pylori in a lot more detail in *Kick Reflux, Heartburn, & GERD in the Nuts* and I don't want to waste a lot of space here. But right here in the book you're reading now, I will cover the complex supplement protocol that seems to be the most effective at wiping out an H. pylori infection. This infection can be difficult to take care of. It's my experience that a few things need to be used in conjunction with each other to have a successful outcome. When fighting H. pylori, even the medical world will use two different antibiotics and a proton pump inhibitor at the same time to wipe them out. The problems with this method are: Not only are you using antibiotics which kill bacteria but still lay the foundation for fungal problems later on, you are also turning off the protective acid barrier and opening the door for any bad guys that want to come in while the acid is shut down. I'm not much of a fan for any strategy that lets every annoying little scumbag in the world of bacteria, fungus, and parasites come on in for a party.

Here are the main players in the natural world that seem to get the best results when used together in an attempt to eradicate H. pylori:

• Zinc
Zinc has the ability to kill H. pylori, specifically liquid zinc in the form of zinc sulphate. This is a great place to start. A company called BodyBio makes a liquid zinc that I like a lot. I've seen people use 15 drops twice a day with pretty good success. Zinc is also believed to be one of the minerals needed to produce your own HCL, so that can be a nice bonus. If you're using HCL supplementation, including zinc in your protocol may be a good idea because doing so will give your body an additional tool it can use to make its own HCL. Empirical Labs makes a digestive enzyme called HCL-Zyme that includes a little bit of zinc. This is a great formula to use when you're trying to increase HCL production.

Along with zinc, it is also popular to use an amino acid, L-Carnisole, for this issue. You can even find "zinc carnisole" manufactured by many companies. I still like to use the liquid zinc even if I'm going to use zinc carnisole. If I use plain L-Carnisole capsules with the liquid zinc, one L-Carnisole capsule twice a day seems to be effective.

• HCL

Since H. pylori are happier in an alkaline environment, increasing stomach acid is always an important step. Not only can H. pylori scarf up all your hydrogen so the body can't make much HCL, they also pee ammonia. Ammonia is an alkaline substance and can alkalize the stomach even further, totally pimping out their pad to optimize life for H. pylori.

• Pyloricin

Pyloricin is an herbal product made by a company called Pharmax. It's available to consumers at many health food stores and online retailers. When you open the bottle and smell the capsules, your reaction will be, "Oh yeah, I wouldn't want to live in a place that smelled like that either, so I imagine this will work nicely." It's not disgusting to take, you're just swallowing capsules. But it does make your pee smell funky so you know it's doing something, right? The word on the street (and the words coming out of my mouth from my experience) is that this product works better than just about anything else out there.

I've seen people take two capsules, three times a day, and work through two bottles and be done. I still use this product in conjunction with other efforts I'm describing here since I don't think any of these supplements would do the job on their own.

• Pepto-Bismol

What? I know, I know. Pepto-Bismol is not very natural. But it's basically just bismuth. Be sure to use the original and not the cherry flavored or any of the other varieties that have extra junk in them. Bismuth is a heavy metal that is found in our bodies already and can be very effective at wiping out bacteria in the stomach. When H. pylori begin to die from the other supplements you are using, they can often clench on to the side of your stomach and create a cramping feeling. It's really not that fun. If you feel this, you can take Pepto-Bismol, which will help finish them off and relieve your cramping faster. (Not to be confused with menstrual cramps, this is not the same thing.) The cramping may still last a while longer, but using the Pepto can reduce the duration of those cramps. Since the active ingredient, bismuth, is a heavy metal, I try not to use Pepto-Bismol for longer than a week to ten days at a time.

So, Pepto-Bismol isn't one that I start off with, but I do recommend having it on hand once you start the rest of this protocol so you can be ready if you experience any stomach cramps.

• Bee Propolis or Mastic Gum

I describe bee propolis and mastic gum together because they work in similar fashions and seem to be the most popular choice. I've never seen anyone with H. pylori use one of these products without improvement, but I've also never seen anyone totally eradicate the problem with one of these supplements and nothing else. I'll explain how they work and you'll understand why. I do, however, feel that they are an excellent part of the arsenal I would use to wipe out H. pylori. I just hear a lot of people suggesting that this is enough to take care of the problem and I don't agree with that at all. That's like thinking that one counseling session is going to straighten out Lindsey

234

Lohan. She could probably use a whole team of counselors; and reading my upcoming book, *Kick Your Crazy in the Nuts,* might be a good place to start.

Back to bee propolis. When a mouse crawls into a beehive, the bees will sting it to death and the mouse invader will be neutralized. Now, if you're a bee, you have a dead and rotting mouse in your house. It's not like the bees can just chuck it out the back door. What they do is cover the mouse in what is called propolis. It basically mummifies the mouse so that it doesn't rot in the hive. That's why bee propolis is used as a natural antibiotic. It goes in and essentially mummifies any bacteria so it can be safely removed from the body. Mastic gum works in the same way. The problem is, these bacteria can crawl up into the mucous lining of the stomach and avoid being swept away in a sticky cocoon. I certainly believe that you can wipe out a percentage of the infection with each dose; but at the rate H. pylori replicate, I think other tools need to be used as well to take care of the whole problem. That's why people seem to see improvements when they use these products, but the problem often multiplies again as soon as they discontinue use.

Since bee propolis or mastic gum also have the ability to wipe out good bacteria, using probiotics for a couple weeks after you are done using the bee propolis or mastic gum may be a good idea. It seems like people do well with two or three capsules of bee propolis or mastic gum twice a day on an empty stomach—first thing when waking up and again right before going to bed.

HCL With A Catabolic Imbalance

With a Catabolic Imbalance, the body will normally send more water to the bowels and less to the kidneys. This can result in bile becoming too thick and sticky to flow properly. Like I talked about earlier in this chapter with loose stool issues, a lack of bile flow can leave the acid product from the stomach un-neutralized. Acid that isn't neutralized with proper bile flow is going to travel quickly through the system so it doesn't burn your intestinal walls. This can result in your sitting on the toilet and shooting off like a rocket. Since that is not beneficial, it is recommended that those with a Catabolic Imbalance use a very low dose of HCL, if they feel like they need to use any at all.

Once the Catabolic Imbalance has improved and you have taken the steps to thin your bile and allow it to flow more freely, you can try to increase your HCL use, if needed. Just keep in mind that if you have plenty of acid coming from the stomach and not enough bile to cool it off, and you continue this behavior for some time, you can create a duodenal ulcer when the acid moves into the duodenum and there is not enough bile dropping down to take care of neutralizing it. With that in mind, I cover creating better bile flow next. Before I get there, let's cover another option you can use until your bile flow improves, if HCL is too strong for you due to a lack of bile flow.

While your Catabolic Imbalance is still strong, you can use apple cider vinegar to improve your digestion. Apple cider vinegar is acidic and a tablespoon toward the end of a meal can help digestion. It's not as acidic as HCL, but it is still something. The real benefit is that apple cider vinegar can be pro-anabolic for most people. That means it can help make you less catabolic while it's helping you digest. Just be sure to get a good apple cider vinegar that contains what they call "The Mother" and they will list that on the label. Bragg makes a good organic apple cider vinegar that I like and can be found in most health food stores. A tablespoon of Swedish bitters toward the end of the meal can be helpful as well, but I see better results with apple cider vinegar for catabolics.

One word of warning: Apple cider vinegar can be harder to neutralize than HCL, even though HCL is more acidic. So, for some catabolics, using apple cider vinegar can create diarrhea as well if you use too much.

Bile Flow

I have thoroughly covered the acid side of digestion, but don't just skip out on the alkaline, bile side of the process. Not only is proper bile flow a key factor in making digestion work, it's also one of the body's main pathways to remove filth. That's why improving bile flow can be such an effective measure when improving nausea issues. I'm not going to go into that here because you will be able to learn more about that when I release *Kick Nausea in the Nuts*. However, if you do have nausea issues, don't be surprised if you see them improve once your bile is flowing better.

Before I talk about supplements that can specifically help bile flow, don't forget that correcting a Catabolic Imbalance, if you have one, is a key move when dealing with bile flow. Any steps you take to improve a Catabolic Imbalance can also help in a big way toward improving bile flow. With this in mind, make your Catabolic Imbalance, if you have one, a priority when it comes to working on this part of digestion.

- Beets and Beet Greens
Beets and beet greens are absolutely the most effective components in improving bile flow, in my opinion. Eating beets and beet greens is okay, but you're going to be eating beets all day, every day, if you want to match the effects you can see from using some concentrated supplement forms. People will often use beet products to help bile flow, but if the product doesn't also contain the beet greens, it's not going to work as effectively.

My favorite product containing beets and beet greens is Beet Flow from Empirical Labs. This product is available to consumers at www.NaturalReference.com. It's a little pricey, but most beet products are.

Most people use Beet Flow at the rate of 2-5 per meal. If you're using Beet Flow, you can do what is called a Beet Flow Flush after you've been using the product with meals for a day or two. I like to see people do this flush at least once, especially if their saliva pH is below 6.5. Low saliva pH can be an indication that the liver is backed up and bile is not flowing well. This flush can really help to get things moving again.

The Beet Flow Flush is like eating a bucket of organic beets and beet greens without having to actually do that. This is an easy cleanse that can help your bile flow better and improve how your lymph is moving. Beet Flow thins the bile and allows it to flow more freely. Improved bile flow will normally result in better liver detoxification. This simply means the liver puts a lot of the body's filth into our bile so it can be removed out the south gate in our stool. That's why it's so important for bile to move properly. If bile is stuck and not flowing, junk is getting backed up in the system. If your saliva pH begins to rise in the next day or so following this flush, or if your stool begins to get darker, you know it worked well. It is acceptable to do this cleanse every week in the beginning, for a few weeks if needed, and again every month or so if your stool starts to get lighter, or if your saliva pH drops below 6.5.

Here's how I do the flush:

- About an hour or so after a meal I take four Beet Flow with water.
- 30 minutes later I take four more.
- 30 minutes later I take four more.

238

▪ 30 minutes later I take four more. If I have the supplement Choline Max, I'll include two only in this dose. (I talk about choline next.)

To recap, I take four Beet Flow capsules every 30 minutes for four doses. I drink water during this time.

And that's it. You're done. Then you can watch your saliva pH the next day or so and if it doesn't come up, you can do the flush again the following week.

This is a very easy flush. It's all about the power of beets moving your bile and helping your liver to function at a higher standard. It's about getting that lymph flowing better so you can remove garbage. It really works unbelievably well for some people. Most people don't really feel different right away but when their self-test numbers start to improve they can see it worked.

If you get hungry or feel uncomfortable during the flush, it's okay to eat a little something in the middle and that won't influence the outcome.

• Choline

The nutrient choline is used to help a person digest fats and is often used in supplement form. Choline is believed to thin bile so it flows better, and possibly even increase bile production. Its use will also alkalize the bloodstream and can be used for those whose self-tests show that their blood appears to be tending too acidic. On the other hand, if your breath rate is below fourteen, your blood may already be tending too alkaline so choline would not be an appropriate choice for you until your breath rate comes up a little.

My favorite choline product is Choline Max from Empirical Labs, only available through a health coach. It's my favorite because it contains ingredients that can help to dilate the gallbladder tube so bile can flow better. Some of the ingredients in Choline Max can be found in coffee suppositories and enemas; and, in a way, it is thought to help pull the bile out of the biliary pathway, almost from the other direction, so to speak. For people whose bile is really stuck, the most effective practice I have seen is using a beet and beet greens supplement along with some coffee suppositories. Choline Max sometimes works as well as a coffee suppository without having to stick something up your butt.

Choline is usually dosed dependent on a person's breath rate. A dose of 1-2 capsules or tablets per meal is ordinarily okay, but only when breath rate stays above fourteen or fifteen. If breath rate drops below that range, choline would need to be reduced or discontinued until breath rate came back up. The reason is that you don't want to further alkalize a bloodstream that is tending too alkaline already; and choline can do just that.

▪ Coffee Enema or Suppository
Coffee enemas can be very effective, but also very messy and little less than fun. A company by the name of RemedyLink, Inc. makes a coffee suppository called Xenaplex. You need to buy it from a health coach, but it is just as effective as a coffee enema, in my opinion. I find that most people don't need to go this route unless their bile is really having a hard time moving, or they are having gallstones or gallbladder issues, indicating that the bile is very stagnant. At that point, a coffee enema or suppository can be a great option.

What If My Gallbladder Was Yanked?

I talked a lot in chapter eight about the function of the gallbladder and how, if people have had gallbladder removal surgery, they're

240

pretty much screwed. But I did shed some light at the end of the "some jackass yanked out my gallbladder" tunnel, and that light was ox bile supplementation. If you have had your gallbladder removed, I recommend returning to chapter eight and reviewing that information to make sure you understand the importance of taking the right steps to create better digestion. I'm adding this topic again in this chapter on digestive supplements so you can review specifics about different ox bile products and methods of using them.

Empirical Labs makes a good ox bile product called Bil-E-Mulsion, but you need a health coach to order it. Just remember what I talked about in chapter eight: You can't take an ox bile product with your food to simulate proper digestion because the bile is alkaline and will neutralize the acid in your stomach, thereby turning off digestion instead of creating it. The trick is to take one or two capsules or tablets away from your meals. If you can put the bile into your intestinal tract between your meals, it can help neutralize any acids that may not have been neutralized during digestion.

I see the most success when people can remember to take ox bile at least two to three hours after they eat (so the food has been digested and has moved out of the stomach), and at least 45-60 minutes before they eat again, so the bile product has time to move through the stomach before the food enters and the stomach acid kicks in. Remember, you don't want the alkaline bile product to neutralize the acid while it's still in the stomach. You want the acid to be able to do its job while it's in the stomach.

Digestive Enzymes

Chapter eight covered why digestive enzymes are important so review that chapter if needed. In the spirit of using chapter twelve as a reference guide while you're still figuring out what supplements are right for you, I will remind you here that to maximize digestion, adults should supplement enzymes any time they are eating food. Some authorities will tell you that enzymes are only needed anytime you eat cooked or processed foods. But since today's food supply doesn't contain the nutrients it once did, it can be a good idea to use enzymes with any type of meal. As you age, your body's stockpile of usable enzymes diminishes. If you don't supply your body with digestive enzymes, your body steals enzymes used for repair and turns them into digestive enzymes, leaving less repairing enzymes for their intended use. Even if someone told me to piss off regarding everything else I said in this book, many readers could see some amazing improvements if they just added digestive enzymes and sea salt.

It's also fun to watch people add enzymes into their diets and have a new ability to eat foods they couldn't eat before. I talked about how some food allergy-like reactions are a result of people missing the enzyme that is needed to process that food. Many lactose intolerance issues can be corrected by simply using enzymes that contain lactase (the enzyme needed to process lactose). These lactose intolerant people were missing just that one necessity that allowed them to cheese it up. This reminds me of the famous quote, "Supplied with the proper tools, your accomplishments may soar far beyond what you ever dreamed." - Bernie Madoff

Note for those with a Catabolic Imbalance: I'm relatively cautious when using digestive enzymes with catabolic individuals. Although enzyme companies recommend digestive enzymes as being harmless, consuming more than is needed for digestion may facilitate connective tissue breakdown in a catabolic person.

Empirical Labs makes a digestive enzyme called Omnizyme that I really like. It's available without a health coach at www.NaturalReference.com. There are other enzymes that can be more powerful in specific situations, but you need a health coach to buy those. Additionally, a health coach will be able to help you determine if a more powerful enzyme is appropriate for you.

Outside of those circumstances, Omnizyme can be a great digestive enzyme.

Sea Salt (Unrefined Salt)

Chapter nine supplied you with information about sea salt. Since this one topic is one of THE most important pieces of information in this book, I cover sea salt again in this digestive supplements chapter. You may come back later and just review the supplements chapters and I want this information to be here for you. I'm pretty much going to tell you the same things about sea salt again, but I'll change the way I say them so you don't yell at me for putting the same paragraph in this book twice. But really take the time to read this again because it's a crucial piece of the puzzle. Sea salt is so important, when it comes to cramps, this book could have been called, "Sea Salt Knocked the Bitch out of Me." Those of you who get the types of cramps that make you want to punch everyone in the mouth know exactly what I'm talking about. Girls becoming meaner during their period is such a lame cliché because most guys couldn't put up with the pain that can come with cramps. But it is amazing to see the number of women who tell me that their bad temper seems to completely leave them once they correct the cramping.

Keep in mind that emotional symptoms around your period occur only for some women. Just like any issue, severity and the variety of symptoms that can accompany that issue can be different for every person. Even if you have no trouble with anger or severe emotional swings during your period, it can be a very real problem for others. This is why sea salt can be so important. Your body needs more resources during your cycle; and if too many resources are being used to carry out the functions of your cycle, that can leave a deficiency in the rest of the body's systems. A lack of minerals can lead to a lack of signals from the body to the brain, which can create emotional symptoms. A good sea salt can help replenish some of these needed minerals so that the body can continue functioning at the same level it does away from your cycle.

Don't forget how the chloride ion found in sea salt is necessary for your body to make its own HCL (stomach acid). Therefore, if your blood pressure is low, a good sea salt can even ensure that your digestion continues to work properly during your cycle. As I said, "Flower of the Ocean" by Celtic Sea Salt is my favorite brand, but don't feel like this is your only option. Any unrefined salt or unrefined sea salt should bring you some benefits. Redmond Real Salt is a popular unrefined salt used by many health coaches. Some feel that, since the sea is polluted, it is better to use a mined salt like Redmond Real Salt. Even if you're out at a restaurant and don't have any sea salt available to you, normal table salt could help you out of a rough spot in your cycle when your body may be screaming for more resources.

CHAPTER THIRTEEN

Supplements For Specific Imbalances

As I go through the imbalances, I list supplements that seem to be beneficial for each imbalance. For some supplements, I add commentary about the key players or mention dosages that I have seen people use successfully. If I don't mention a dose, that supplement may be a little too complicated to suggest a dose without seeing your specific chemistry. You may need to follow the label (and regrettably telling someone to follow the label is less than helpful, since what is on the label is regulated more by legal concerns than reasonableness or health concerns) or find a health coach who can look at your chemistry and help you figure out how much to use and when. Just be sure to understand that you are responsible for your own health and you have to decide what dosage is best for you. After you begin using a supplement, don't forget how important it is to continue to run your self-tests and monitor your numbers. Monitoring your numbers can help guide you in the dose you are using for many supplements, once you understand how a supplement can affect your body chemistry.

If you are currently working with health care professionals, you should always let them know what you are considering using just to make sure it is not contradicting anything they have you using already. Below, I'm not making any suggestions to you because I don't know you. You do remember that you only bought my book and we're not really talking, right? So, I couldn't possibly have a clue what your chemistry is or how much of each supplement you should take and when. I'm sure you see that would be a ridiculous assumption. I'm just going to list amounts that I have seen people use with success.

I will also list supplements that are contraindicated for each imbalance. This is very important to pay attention to because you don't want to try to fix one imbalance and simultaneously make another imbalance that showed up on your *Imbalance Guide* worse. For example, you may see that L-Glutamine can help a Catabolic Imbalance so you decide to use it since your Catabolic Imbalance was so strong. But L-Glutamine is contraindicated for an Electrolyte Excess Imbalance, so if you also showed an Electrolyte Excess Imbalance, L-Glutamine could actually exacerbate that issue. Pay attention to what you're doing and, before you use a supplement to improve one imbalance, make sure it is not listed under the "avoid" section of another imbalance that showed up on your *Imbalance Guide*. This is one of the reasons why it can be so beneficial to employ the help of professional health coaches who understand these principles. Not only have they studied these principles extensively, they have also seen these fundamentals work, first hand, in their clients' efforts, so they can help you eliminate time-wasting moves.

For those of you not working with a health coach, I list which supplements are available to consumers and which ones need to be purchased through a health coach. I try to list the supplements in order of their effectiveness, in relation to my experience and knowledge. Just remember, the most "effective" supplements according my experience may not bring you the best results. You may do better with something that I see work only occasionally. I find it's best to assume that, since you're a human, you will operate like most other humans with similar imbalances. The trick is to keep in mind that we really are all different in one way or another so don't walk through this process like a zombie. Really pay attention to what you're doing, how you're feeling, and most importantly, where your numbers are going. By keeping charts of your progress, you can get a visual overview of how you are doing.

The biggest mistake I see consumers make when it comes to supplements is that they will buy a supplement because their friend tells them it is good for a specific symptom—they'll start to use it and they will feel better. "Yay! I found something that works," they tell themselves. They will then continue to use this supplement FOREVER! No matter what. Even if the symptom comes back or gets worse, they will continue to use that supplement because they think, "Well, this helped me before so it must be something else that is causing the problem or the problem must just be escalating and now I need to add something else too." Don't do that. I've smacked people in the head for less than that. Watch your numbers, see the patterns, and adjust what you're doing accordingly. I can't emphasize that enough.

Before I get to the imbalances, my final point is this: Under some imbalances I will list quite a few supplements that may help that imbalance. That does not mean that you should use all of those supplements just because that imbalance showed up on your *Imbalance Guide*. Unless your imbalance appears to be very strong, you might want to start with just one or two of the supplements listed under a given imbalance and then see if your self-testing numbers improve, indicating the imbalance is improving. If you don't see improvement, it might be time to add another supplement that is listed as beneficial under that imbalance.

It's nice to have a variety to choose from, since you may be experiencing more than one imbalance at one time. Let's say that you show Catabolic and Electrolyte Excess Imbalances on your *Imbalance Guide*. You may see that L-Glutamine could help your Catabolic Imbalance, but it's contraindicated for your Electrolyte Excess Imbalance. In this scenario, you could maybe use Sterols instead of L-Glutamine since Sterols are listed as beneficial under Catabolic and Electrolyte Excess.

Just pay attention to what you're doing and start slow and easy instead of throwing fifteen new supplements into your body at once.

My only exception to this rule is if you are looking at digestive issues that need attention. When there are digestive issues, and it's likely there will be for most people dealing with menstrual cramps, you need to address all aspects of digestion. Don't just start by using HCL and think you can add Beet Flow in later. You need to address the lack of acid, and use the Beet Flow to help bile flow correctly. You also need to make sure you are using some type of digestive enzyme to fully improve digestive issues. With this understanding, it's simple to see that the "start off slowly" approach does not apply to digestion. You still want to start off slowly with your quantities and build your way up, but when it comes to digestion, you really want to hit all the angles from the beginning.

Imbalance - Electrolyte Deficiency

The most important factors with an Electrolyte Deficiency Imbalance are correcting digestion and adding more unrefined salt. Try to make these your priorities and add other supplements from below as secondary tools.

Often Used with this Imbalance
- Electrolyte Deficiency from Empirical Labs - Health coach required.
- L-Glutamine - An amino acid - Don't use with an Anabolic Imbalance. L-Glutamine can be bought in powder or capsule form in just about any health food store. It's a good idea to use powder since many people use doses of a full teaspoon at a time. You would need to take a lot of capsules to equal one teaspoon. If you become constipated while using L-Glutamine, you could be using too much and may need to reduce your dose.

248

- Cal-Amo from Standard Process - Health coach required - Avoid with an Acid Imbalance. (Only take with breakfast and/or lunch.)
- L-Tyrosine - An amino acid - Good for Parasympathetic or Fat Burner Imbalances - Avoid with Catabolic or Sympathetic Imbalances. (Avoid at night.)
- Zinc - Keep dose low with an Anabolic Imbalance.

<u>Avoid</u>
- Drinking too much water or drinking distilled water
- Vitamin E
- Sterols from Empirical Labs
- L-Arginine - An amino acid

Imbalance - Electrolyte Excess

Use water as a supplement. If you have an Electrolyte Excess Imbalance, odds are great that you are not drinking enough water. If you also have a Catabolic Imbalance, and drinking more water gives you diarrhea, first improve your Catabolic Imbalance and then you may be able to increase your water intake, without inducing a loose stool.

<u>Often Used with this Imbalance</u>
- L-Arginine - An amino acid - Avoid with an Anabolic Imbalance. (Best taken before bed)
- Arginex from Standard Process - Health coach required.
- L-Taurine - An amino acid - Avoid with a Catabolic Imbalance. (Best taken in the morning, and near lunch.)
- Vitamin E - Avoid with an Anabolic Imbalance. (Best taken with dinner.)
- Electrolyte Excess from Empirical Labs - Health coach required.
- Cardio VH from Empirical Labs - Health coach required.

- Sterols from Empirical Labs - Health coach required. (Best taken with dinner.)

Avoid
- Vitamin D3
- L-Glutamine - An amino acid

Imbalance - Anabolic

Often Used with this Imbalance
- Vitamin B12 - Can also help the body burn fat. (Best taken with breakfast and/or lunch. Avoid at night.)
- Magnesium (Best taken with breakfast and/or lunch. Avoid at night.)
- Anabolic from Empirical Labs - Health coach required. (Best taken with breakfast and/or lunch. Avoid at night.)
- Mito NRG from Empirical Labs - Health coach required. (Best taken with breakfast and/or lunch. Avoid at night.)
- Vitamin A (Best taken with breakfast and/or lunch. Avoid at night.)
- L-Tyrosine - An amino acid. (Best taken with breakfast and/or lunch. Avoid at night.)
- Flax seed oil - Pearl form or gelcap is best. (Best taken with breakfast and/or lunch. Avoid at night.)
- Cal-Amo from Standard Process - Health coach required - Avoid with an Acid Imbalance. (Best taken with breakfast and/or lunch. Avoid at night.)

Avoid
- L-Glutamine - An amino acid
- L-Arginine - An amino acid
- Vitamin E
- Potassium Citrate

Imbalance - Catabolic

Don't forget about poached or soft boiled eggs with this imbalance. Any type of egg where the yolk is still runny can benefit a Catabolic Imbalance. Be sure to use hormone-free eggs. Real butter and coconut oil can also almost be considered to create supplement-like, beneficial results for some people with a Catabolic Imbalance.

Often Used with this Imbalance

- L-Glutamine - An amino acid - Avoid with an Electrolyte Excess Imbalance. (Best taken after dinner, before bed, away from food.)
- L-Arginine - An amino acid - Avoid with an Electrolyte Deficiency Imbalance. (Best taken after dinner, before bed.)
- Sterols from Empirical Labs - Health coach required - Avoid with an Electrolyte Deficiency Imbalance. (Best taken with dinner.)
- Catabolic from Empirical Labs - Health coach required. (Best taken with dinner.)
- Vitamin E - Avoid with an Electrolyte Deficiency Imbalance. (Best taken with dinner, or before bed.)
- Potassium Citrate
- HMB (Best taken with dinner.)
- Glucosomine Sulfate - Great for joint pain when dealing with a Catabolic Imbalance. (Best taken with dinner.)
- Apple Cider Vinegar - A tablespoon with meals can aid digestion. Even just adding some apple cider vinegar to water that you drink throughout the day can be beneficial to a catabolic. Be cautious using apple cider vinegar, as it can create loose stool issues if your bile is not flowing properly.

Avoid
- Fatty acids like fish or flax seed oil

251

- L-Tyrosine - An amino acid
- Magnesium
- L-Taurine - An amino acid

Imbalance - Tricarb Fast Oxidizer (Carb Burner)

Often Used with this Imbalance
- Vitamin B12 - Can help move fat into the mitochondria to be burned for fuel. (Best taken with breakfast and/or lunch. Avoid at night.)
- Gluco+ from Empirical Labs - Health coach required.
- Vitamin B5 - Also great for breakouts if the person is not processing fats correctly - Limit use with an Anabolic Imbalance. (Best taken at night.)
- Mito NRG from Empirical Labs - Health coach required. (Best taken with breakfast and/or lunch. Avoid at night.)
- L-Glutamine - An amino acid - Avoid with Anabolic or Electzolyte Excess Imbalances.

Avoid
- Vitamin D3
- L-Histadine - An amino acid
- Vitamin E

Imbalance - Beta Slow Oxidizer (Fat Burner)

Often Used with this Imbalance
- Lipid+ from Empirical Labs - Health coach required - (Best taken with breakfast. Avoid at night)
- Banaba Chrome from Empirical Labs - Health coach required - Great for weight loss. (Best taken with lunch and dinner)
- Magnesium Malate - Avoid with a Catabolic Imbalance. (Best taken with breakfast. Avoid at night)
- Vitamin A - Limit with a Catabolic Imbalance.

- L-Taurine - An amino acid - Avoid with Electrolyte Deficiency or Catabolic Imbalances.
- Folic Acid - Limit with an Anabolic Imbalance.

Avoid
- Vitamin B5

Imbalance - Parasympathetic

This is the imbalance where allergies normally live. I won't explain allergies here, but I will cover them in great detail when I release *Kick Allergies in the Nuts*. There are other imbalances that would normally take precedence over this imbalance, but if allergies are driving you up the wall at any particular time, you might want to increase some of the supplements outlined here during that bout to try to improve your allergies. If you have an Electrolyte Deficiency Imbalance, correcting that will often help this imbalance as well. Improving digestion can play a big role in improving this imbalance.

Often Used with this Imbalance
- L-Phenylalanine - An amino acid - Good for an Anabolic Imbalance as well - Avoid with Catabolic or Sympathetic Imbalances. Most people with allergies love this stuff. Single amino acids have the ability to correct problems and also induce problems if not used carefully. For this reason, more than casual attention needs to be given to monitoring where your numbers are; see if your numbers on the *Data Tracking Sheet* have moved to a range that would allow you to reduce the use of any specific amino acid. (Best taken with or breakfast and/or lunch. Avoid at night.)
- Auto P from Empirical Labs - Health coach required - Great for allergies.
- L-Glutamine - An amino acid - Avoid with Anabolic or Electrolyte Excess Imbalances. (Best taken after dinner, before bed, away from food.)

- Vitamin B5 - Also great for breakouts if the person is having trouble processing fats correctly - Limit use with an Anabolic Imbalance.
- Magnesium Chloride - Great for allergies - Avoid with a Catabolic Imbalance. (Best taken with breakfast and/or lunch. Avoid at night.)
- Mito NRG from Empirical Labs - Health coach required - Avoid with a Catabolic Imbalance. (Best taken with breakfast and/or lunch. Avoid at night.)
- L-Tyrosine - An amino acid. If you are taking L-Phenylalanine, then L-Tyrosine is not needed since L-Phenylalanine turns into L-Tyrosine. (Best taken with or breakfast and/or lunch. Avoid at night.)

Avoid
- Vitamin B6
- L-Histadine - An amino acid
- Vitamin D3
- Potassium Citrate

Imbalance - Sympathetic

Often Used with this Imbalance
- Manganese - Limit with a Catabolic Imbalance. (Best taken with breakfast and/or lunch. Avoid at night.)
- Vitamin E - Avoid with Electrolyte Deficiency or Anabolic Imbalances. (Best taken with dinner.)
- Auto S from Empirical Labs - Health coach required.
- L-Arginine - An amino acid - Avoid with Electrolyte Deficiency or Anabolic Imbalances. (Best taken at night.)
- L-Taurine - An amino acid - Avoid with Electrolyte Deficiency or Catabolic Imbalances. (Best taken with breakfast and/or lunch. Avoid at night.)

Avoid

- L-Phenylalanine - An amino acid
- L-Tyrosine - An amino acid
- Magnesium Chloride
- Vitamin B5

Imbalance - Tending To Acidosis

Often Used with this Imbalance

- Choline Max from Empirical Labs - Health coach required.
- Choline - Nutrient in the B vitamin family.

Avoid

- Ammonium Phosphate from Empirical Labs
- Cal-Amo from Standard Process

Imbalance - Tending To Alkalosis

Often Used with this Imbalance

- Ammonium Phosphate from Empirical Labs - Health coach required. (Best taken with breakfast and/or lunch. Avoid at night.)
- Cal-Amo from Standard Process - Health coach required. (Best taken with breakfast and/or lunch. Avoid at night.)

Avoid

- Alkalizing water
- Alkalizing supplements
- L-Arginine - An amino acid

Finding A Qualified Health Coach In Your Area

If you would like to find a qualified health coach who can help you with some of these supplement choices, go to www.OurCoaltion.org and fill out the "Find a Health Coach" form. The Coalition will locate a health coach in your area who will contact you directly.

CHAPTER FOURTEEN

A Healthy Body In An Unhealthy World

Nobody can avoid everything that is bad for the human body. It's just not possible in the world we live in. Even if you cancel your DirecTV subscription, fire your dog walker, and move out into the woods, you can still have a bird fly over and poop in your mouth while you're sunbathing next to a natural stream. The trick is not to try to eliminate every toxin, chemical and pollutant from entering your body, but instead, to put your body in a position where it can have an easier time of removing those toxins. That's the whole point in improving the "flow" of the body and balancing the systems that make it all work.

While you're helping your body perform at a higher level, the next goal is to merely learn about the facets of your life that are contributing to your body's toxic load, then get rid of the ones that are the easiest for you to eliminate. Don't feel like you need to run in horror from every environmental or household pollutant within a thirty mile radius or you're going to be doing some Forrest Gump-type running. However, if there are factors in your life that are easy for you to change, go ahead and change them. That will be one less irritant that your body has to deal with—one less task that it needs to take care of before it can move on to more important bodily processes.

It's my view that the body was designed to handle some of this junk. Worrying about every possible toxin is just going to create more stress, more harmful chemicals that accompany that stress, and more work for your body to deal with. Crimeny Pete! Chill out and enjoy your life. I don't think your priority should be to eliminate every toxin from your little world in the next forty-eight hours. Simply understanding how these toxins get into your body can be enough to let you begin removing them little by little. Once the load coming in begins to decrease, it will be easier for your body to deal with any toxins that remain.

In this chapter, I also talk about items that many people feel are healthy solutions. I explain why these people are idiots. They may not truly be idiots—they may just be mislead—but I'm going to call them idiots anyway, just because it's faster and easier. Bear in mind that almost every product, method or idea out there could benefit *somebody*. I think there are very few ideas that are completely invalid for the entire population. I just get annoyed when people try to push their products on everyone and market their products as if they are the solution to every human ailment available today. I feel strongly that there is no such product; a lot of it has to do with what happens to be popular at any given moment. I mean, now it seems popular to watch shows about people getting screamed at in a kitchen. Who saw that coming?

Before I dive into this chapter, I'd like to pause and reflect on a few things:

- Don't treat your symptoms and don't use symptoms to label yourself with an imbalance.
- Get help. This work can get very complicated. If you run into trouble, find a health coach in your area who can help you.
- I just want to point out that I've completed more than thirteen chapters of this book without once making fun of Paris Hilton or Snookie. Sometimes, I amaze even myself.

Water

Water is a pretty big deal when discussing the toxicity level in a human body. After all, water is one of the biggest components that allows the human body to wash toxins out. The body is 70% water and is based on aqueous chemistry; it doesn't work too well without the aqueous. If you're not drinking enough water, you're trying to wash your windows with mud. I did explain earlier how those with low mineral levels normally need to qualify before they can increase their water intake. They need to qualify to drink more water by increasing their mineral levels, so don't ignore that suggestion. Still, since the body uses water to help remove junk, don't you think it would be a good idea to drink water that is not filled with junk in the first place? If your car is covered in dirt, does it make sense to wash it off with water that was filled with smashed up chocolate chip cookies? Maybe if you wanted all the kids in your neighborhood licking your car, but that's weird and I'm pretty sure you would end up with your face on some warning fliers around town. My point is, your car wouldn't get cleaner; you would just be replacing one layer of junk with another layer of junk.

Chemicals In Tap Water

I was at my brother's house in Florida this summer when we decided to use his pool testing kit to look at his tap water. We tested both his pool and the water from the tap in his kitchen. We both sort of freaked when we saw that there was more chlorine in his tap water than in his pool! Seriously?! My brother freaked because he thought, "Man, I must really need more chlorine in my pool," and ran out to his shed to add more. But his pool wasn't green with algae and it became clear the next day, as all of our eyes were burning in the pool during a game of paddle ball, that he really didn't need more chlorine in his pool—he needed less in his tap water.

Most city water treatment plants use both chlorine and fluoride to treat the water. Both of these chemicals are harmful to the human body in their own right. An immediate impact these chemicals can have on the body is their ability to "displace" iodine from the body. I say "displace" because that is how most researchers view what chlorine and fluoride are doing to iodine levels in the body. Though iodine levels do normally go down if consuming chlorine and fluoride laden water, I view this another way: Iodine acts as a disperser in the body. It disperses toxins so they can be removed from the system. The body views chlorine and fluoride as toxins. (Yes, I know your dentist told you fluoride was good for your teeth, but what he didn't tell you is that it is not good for your body... oops. He will also tell you mercury in your mouth isn't dangerous.) Therefore, iodine is used to help disperse these toxins. In essence, these chemicals are stripping, or displacing, the iodine from the system, but it makes more sense to view this as the body is just using up its iodine to deal with this problem.

It is widely accepted that iodine is required for proper thyroid function, and thyroid "conditions" have been on the rise in the past decade or so. Although I feel that the rise of this epidemic has more to do with the rise in popularity of prescribing thyroid medications, it could also be partially due to the fact that cities are using more and more chemicals to treat our water. It is also important to consider that iodine is a mineral that can be difficult for some people to absorb. Some minerals are easier to absorb than others and come into the system even if the system is imbalanced. Iodine, on the other hand, requires a more balanced pH in the system in order to be absorbed properly. That's why giving iodine to patients with thyroid issues will often bring no result. You can dump all the iodine you want into a person, but if it can't be absorbed, it's not going to help. This is why the medical world has shifted to using drugs in most thyroid cases.

The significance of this, in reference to water, is understanding that if people already have a low level of iodine, you can see how drinking tap water filled with chlorine or fluoride could really do a number on their iodine levels. Crazy to see how just drinking tap water could result in a thyroid issue, right? Yet, understanding the science makes it hard to argue.

Most filter pitchers filter the water through carbon and do very little to remove these chemicals from your tap. When it comes to filters, I like the good reverse osmosis filters that can be installed under your sink the best, but even these filters can remove good minerals while they're removing the bad stuff. If you use a reverse osmosis filter, it's a good idea to add mineral drops back into your water. The company, Trace Minerals Research, makes a product called Concentrace Trace Mineral Drops. It's sold at most health food stores. Adding just three or four drops per glass of water can replenish minerals that may have been stripped during the filtration process. Of course, if you have high blood pressure, you would cut that dosage in half.

Spring water is the best option, but it can be costly to buy. I don't really like the idea of distilled water for most people because it is void of any mineral whatsoever, and can wash away more mineral than spring water might. For some people, merely getting any form of water into them is going to be beneficial, so again, I don't want to split hairs with water for some. But since I'm talking about ways to reduce the intake of toxic substances, the type of water can be important.

Shower Filters

Now that you understand the trouble that chlorine can cause, let's hit the showers because most of us don't think about how the water we bathe in can affect our bodies. It's true that most of us don't drink the water coming out of the showerhead while we're washing our hair, but we do continue to breath while we're showering. When that hot water turns into mist and steam, it still contains all the chemicals that are in that water. As we breathe this steam in, those chemicals come into our lungs and can make it into our bloodstream even faster than if we were drinking the water. In a way, this could make the need to filter our shower water even more important than filtering the water we're drinking. Since this water has a faster path to make it to your bloodstream, it can be a good idea to do something to remove the chlorine from this source.

This is a pretty easy fix and I have had a lot of people tell me how much better they started feeling after they added a shower filter. I myself was getting extremely tired after my showers and the only thought I could come up with was, "How long was I in there?!" I never considered that the steam in my shower was filling my lungs with chemicals that my body was scrambling to figure out how to remove. You can buy a shower filter for about $40 at most health food stores. You just screw it onto the shower's water source between the pipe coming out of the wall and the shower head itself and you're done. You can even buy replacement filters for less so you don't have to buy a new filter system every time.

These shower filters usually use carbon to filter the water through, and we already know how that won't remove enough chlorine and fluoride to make water suitable for drinking. In this regard, we know these shower filters are not likely removing all the chemicals from the water. But for such an easy and inexpensive step to take, you can at least reduce the amount chemicals in your showering experience. For a lot of people, this simple step can really reduce the load on their bodies and bring some relief.

Microwaves

Much of this book has been about correcting issues to allow your body to use the food you're eating and also improve its ability to remove junk and synthetic substances that the body can't process. That's why microwaves are an important topic. If you're going to correct your digestion so that you can actually pull the nutrients out of the food you eat, the food you eat should be something that your body can use. The way that microwaves heat food is a process that changes the molecular structure of the food it is heating in order to create the friction that makes it hot. When you change the molecular structure of a natural food, it becomes unrecognizable to the body and the body cannot process it correctly.

Is it easier to heat something up in the microwave? Of course it is. But you need to understand; anything you eat that has been heated by a microwave not only loses its nutritional value to the body, but also now becomes a problem that the body has to deal with. To deal with it, the body often has to strip nutrients from its reserves to help take care of the problem created by your microwaved burrito. By eating food cooked in a microwave, you can be losing nutrients instead of adding them. It will take you longer to prepare your food without a microwave, but it will be time that you save in the long run by reducing the number of doctor and hospital visits you need to make. I just use my microwave as a very fancy clock.

If you're still skeptical and you're thinking, "Okay Tony, I'll fix my digestion, but why ya gotta mess with my Hot Pockets?" I'll give you a little experiment. Go down to Home Depot and buy two identical potted plants. Name one plant "Ricky" and the other one "Reject Bastard-Child." I guess you can pick your own names if you want. In any case, take them home and put them in the same light. Water one plant with normal water, and the other plant with water that has been microwaved. Don't pour the hot water in the plant because obviously that won't go well. Just microwave some water and let it cool to room temperature before you water with it.

At the end of your experiment, I think you will find that one plant is happy, while the other plant has earned the name I suggested. Microwaves can even change the structure of water and turn it into an evil substance. Just imagine what it can do to the food you are putting in your mouth.

What Am I Cooking In?

To keep this brief, understand that what you cook with counts. If you're cooking in plastics, aluminum, or typical "non-stick" cookware, some of these poisons are off-gassing into your food, and into your body. This creates another toxin that your body has to deal with. Some of these heavy metal toxins don't have an exit strategy in the body and can accumulate and cause all types of trouble. Glass is always safe to cook with or drink out of, stainless steel is rarely suspect. Enamel cookware is also considered to be safer than most non-stick cookware.

What's In My Mouth?

The medical field is not the only world that practically gives us a "daily allowance" of toxins. We learned in the middle of the 18th century that mercury is poison and nothing has changed since—mercury is still poison. After the dentist finishes putting mercury into someone's teeth, he takes what is left over and puts it in a special container marked "hazardous materials." That container then goes into another container marked "hazardous materials." Next, a little truck that has the special markings and permits required to haul hazardous materials comes and picks up that mercury from the dentist's office. And of course the ADA doctors will still tell you it's safe to put mercury in your mouth and let it seep into your head 24 hours a day. Dental work that is toxic, medications that are toxic, with all this disclosure I feel like I'm breaking the news to Punky Brewster that there is no Easter Bunny.

Smoking

Smoking? Seriously? I don't really need to explain this, do I? I think you understand that you'll need to stop smoking to have any chance of improving your health. People think that smoking just affects the lungs, but it also puts a lot of tar and chemicals in the body that need to be filtered out by the liver. The two most important factors in health, in my opinion, are digestion and liver function. We aren't what we eat—we are what we can assimilate and what we can't remove. If your liver is overwhelmed, the body is having a hard time removing all the junk that should be removed. If it can't be removed, it will be stored in joints, tissues, or fat cells.

Here's the good news: The people who have a difficult time trying to quit smoking are almost always people with a low mineral content. The tar and the chemicals thicken blood and constrict the vascular system to raise blood pressure. So, when people with no mineral identity try to quit, it can sometimes be hard for them because smoking was helping to lift their blood pressure. If you are a smoker and your *Imbalance Guide* shows that you may be dealing with an Electrolyte Deficiency Imbalance, this is a great indication that losing the smokes might be a whole lot easier if you can improve this imbalance. You're still going to have to want to quit. It's not going to be magic, but it will make it physiologically easier. Understanding how the body works can change the viewpoint of choices that we make in our lives. This new understanding can reveal that a bad habit could actually be a form of self-medication. The exciting part is that the bad habit is easier to get rid of when it no longer represents the only choice for the "medication." To learn more, you will soon be able to check out *Kick Smoking in the Nuts.*

Soda

Soft drinks are just a transport system for artificial sweeteners and chemicals that your body can't process. The worst part is that they also contain phosphates that have been proven to block your body's ability to assimilate nutrients. So, basically, any food that you eat along with a diet soda is not being assimilated optimally by your body. Incredible, isn't it? That's most of the country. It starts to give you some clues why so many in this country are overweight with diabetes, heart disease or cancer. Our bodies aren't getting the nutrients they need to function properly.

Soda can be very hard to quit for some people. You can actually get withdrawal symptoms because the chemicals act like a drug. But once you get past eight or nine days without any soda at all, it will be much easier to quit drinking it completely. Your body will start to forget that it can use those chemicals and sweeteners to thicken your blood—and your cravings can stop altogether.

Most people think that they're making the healthy choice by drinking diet. In my opinion, the only ingest-able substance that you can put in your body that is worse for you than diet soda is a jelly doughnut, and that's only because it's fried. The artificial sweeteners that they use in diet soda are directly linked to so many brain and mental issues that they can't even keep up. Once they get past the initial difficult week of giving up soda, most of my clients lose at least five pounds; and nearly half of their nagging symptoms simply go away.

Just like smoking, those with a low mineral content in their bodies seem to love soda the most, and have the hardest time giving it up. Soda has syrup in it that makes it thicker so the taste sticks on the tongue longer. This syrup also makes your blood thicker and raises your blood pressure. This is one of the reasons people crave it so much and have a hard time quitting. The body can use it to thicken your blood and buffer low salts and sugars.

When many companies ship the concentrated syrup that goes into soda to give it that flavor and texture people can't seem to live without, the companies actually have to post a "Transporting Hazardous Substance" sign on their trucks. And we just dilute this stuff with some carbonated water and drink it? Amazing.

Removing soda from your diet will better help you digest your food, use the nutrients in that food, and can help every aspect of your body. For many people, nothing in this book will improve their health more than losing the soda. When you're drinking soda, not only are you bringing in junk, you're also *not* drinking water... the thing your body really needs.

Artificial Sweeteners

Just about anytime you see "Sugar Free" on a package, you can almost guarantee it's going to have some type of artificial sweetener in it. That's how it still tastes good even though they took all the sugar out. The problem is that these artificial sweeteners are just that: ARTIFICIAL. Some artificial sweeteners market themselves as a natural sweetener and say that they are "made from sugar." That is crap. They are just as bad for you as Sweet'N Low. Because it's artificial, the body can't recognize it and process it properly. Now, it just becomes a toxin that the body has to deal with.

There are also a lot of products out now that are sweetened with agave and honey and such. These are still high in sugars and carbs, but they are natural and better than using an artificial sweetener or refined sugar. I don't view these products as toxic, but since they can spike insulin levels just like sugar can, I try to avoid them. Inositol, inulin, xylitol, and lo han guo are not horrible. Xylitol comes from either corn or birch trees. I'm not much of a fan of anything that comes from corn, so I prefer to use the variety that comes from birch trees, if I use it at all. I'm not a fan of sucralose.

The only sweetener that I honestly view as healthy is stevia. It's just an herb and doesn't have any affect on insulin levels. Stevia is pro-anabolic, so I don't recommend any severe anabolics using large amounts of stevia. But once you improve an anabolic imbalance, introducing small amounts of stevia would likely be okay.

I will be honest, however, and tell you that no one in their right mind could possibly just start using stevia. Disgusting. But here's the trick, and trust me, I have not had one single person who actually followed through with this who didn't say, "Holy cow, you're right, I really like it!" The weird thing is that they all said, "Holy Cow." Weird, huh? Anyway, you can't just start using stevia when your body is used to sugar and artificial sweeteners. The trick is to use whatever you use now, and add just a little bit of stevia. You won't even taste it at first. Then, the next time, you add a little more stevia until you have it at about half and half. Then, you just start using less of your sweetener until it's gone. By that time, your taste buds will have changed and you will have acquired a taste for stevia. Just like you acquired a taste for me. Remember how you used to want to punch me in the face at the beginning of this book, but now I'm just cute? Stevia is just like that. After you get used to it, you will like it. My advice is to get the flavored drops they sell at most health food stores so you get a little bonus flavor.

Antibiotics

Antibiotics don't just break apart the bad bacteria in your body; they also break apart all the good bacteria that live in your intestines. These good bacteria do these good things: Help with digestion, control infestation from yeast and bad bacteria like candida, make the B vitamins we need, and help clean putrefied fecal matter off of colon walls. When we take antibiotics and wipe out all the good bacteria along with the bad, we need to replace the good bacteria with probiotics. Yet our doctors don't normally teach us how to do this.

Here's another issue many people, like myself, have with antibiotics: Many antibiotics are actually made from fungus. When you use these antibiotics to kill a bacterial or viral problem, you're actually setting up the terrain of the body in a way that allows fungal problems to flourish. Imagine you have a garden and weeds are taking over in a big way. Would you try to eliminate those weeds by planting new weeds that were designed to kill the original weeds? That sentence alone sounds horribly dumb just from the number of times "weeds" showed up. If the sentence sounds stupid, obviously the idea is not that brilliant. If you want to get rid of a problem, it might be a good idea to use a method that isn't going to end up creating another problem.

268

Flu Shots

Ignorant.

Alkalizing Water And Water Filters

I talked a lot in this book about how most of the "alkalizing" information in the marketplace today is a heaping pile of fiction. But I want to cover this again here because the alkaline waters and the multilevel companies that sell the $3000-$5000 alkalizing water filters are very popular. You've probably seen a lot of testimonials or maybe even your friend improved his health issues by paying more for a water filter than he spent on his wife's engagement ring. Since the hype can suck you in, I want to break down how this can be misleading.

The first step in digging through this dung is to remember that some individuals have an Acid Imbalance. Their blood is tending toward being too acid. If this imbalance showed up on your *Imbalance Guide*, one of these alkalizing water filters could certainly help you feel better if it was pushing your blood to a more balanced state. You would know if it was working or not if your breath rate started to come down. In this scenario, you would start to feel better and you would tell all of your friends it was because of the "magic water" that was coming out of your water filter and you're so excited because you only have sixty-three more monthly payments before it is paid off.

Let's not stop there. To a lot of my clients, I will hold up a bottle and say, "Have you heard of this? It's called WATER!" because it's so obvious that they're not drinking any. Water is one of the most important components to our health and yet so few people drink enough to help their bodies wash out all the junk. They think that if they're drinking a soda or coffee, that's enough. "It has water in it," they tell me. But soda and coffee, or even sport drinks, are hardly a replacement for water. None of those beverages has the ability to truly hydrate the cells like water can. Most of those

269

drinks just introduce more junk into the body rather than giving your body what it needs to wash junk out. But tell me this: If a guy pays $3000 for a water filter, do you think he might drink some water? You bet he will! He'll probably go fill up a glass every time he opens his checkbook or checks his bank statement. "Where the hell did all my money go? Oh yeah, I guess I should go get a glass of water."

When you take a person who hasn't been drinking any water, and you start getting some H2O down his gullet, that can often be enough to turn his whole world around. You start to hydrate the body; you start to clear out some junk. Pounds get dropped, joints become more flexible, all sorts of happy stuff can happen—just by adding some water. Too bad he could have done the same thing with a ninety-nine cent jug of spring water.

I'll call this water filter-mortgaging consumer "Bill." Bill tells his friend Tanya about this filter and talks her into buying too. (Certainly this is just about her health and has nothing to do with the fact that Bill will be making money off of Tanya's purchase.) But Tanya starts to feel worse. She's exhausted and finds it easier to just sit on the couch all day. If you checked Tanya's breath rate you might see that it's around eight. With a breath rate that low, it could be that Tanya's blood is leaning too alkaline and this alkalizing water is pushing that imbalance further into the abyss.

Since Tanya hears testimonial after testimonial from people who have improved their health by drinking this water, she thinks it must be something else that is bringing her down. It can't be the water because every multilevel marketing meeting she goes to plays loud music and people dance around because they feel so good. Meanwhile, Tanya's blood is so alkaline that oxygen can't get down to the tissues and she just wants to lay down on the floor until they turn off the Macarena.

When deciding if alkalizing water is right for you, it's crucial to look at breath rate and understand if your blood could benefit from drinking this water or if it's just going to make you worse. Even if you do have an Acid Imbalance, and drinking alkaline water could benefit you, be sure to continue to check your breath rate for improvement. You don't want to correct an Acid Imbalance so well that you create an Alkaline Imbalance. Monitoring yourself and your numbers is what this type of health movement is all about. It's not about finding something that makes you feel better and using that product until you die. It's about using something until your body is balanced and then reducing it until you don't need it anymore.

As a side note, remember that the first thing that water hits is your stomach. If you're drinking alkaline water with your food, that alkalinity is going to reduce stomach acid levels that may already be too low.

What About Meat?

I think I get this question more often than just about any other. Is meat healthy? So here's the breakdown:

Chemicals, Hormones And Antibiotics

If you're buying meat at your local grocery store or you're eating at the average restaurant, or just about any fast food place, you're paying for junk meat that was mass-produced. When farmers mass produce in this manner, they often keep the animals in small cages and feed them the cheapest type of food they can come up with so they can make a profit. Keep in mind this farmer has a competitor down the street trying to sell meat to the same large fast food corporation cheaper, and the bean counters on Wall Street are going to tell the corporation to buy the cheaper product with no idea how it became cheaper or where the quality went. Often times, these animals are eating foods that their stomachs were not even designed to eat. The result from this upbringing is frequent illness and a lot of dying animals—animals that could have been sold to make a profit. So what does Mr. Farmer do?

271

He pumps the animals full of antibiotics, drugs and other chemicals to keep them alive long enough to reach a size that will make them profitable.

If you pump a cow or a chicken full of drugs and antibiotics, they don't just poop that out at the end of the day. Those drugs go into their tissues and guess where those tissues end up... yes, right in your cheeseburger. That's why the antibiotic wonder drugs of 30 years ago are beginning to work less and less. We all take in such a small dose of antibiotics on a daily basis through the animal protein we eat that the bad bugs (little bastards that invade our bodies and cause havoc) build up a tolerance to these drugs until they are no longer effective. So, is meat bad? If this is the meat you're eating, yes it is.

Digesting Meat

Another problem with meat is that well over half of the population doesn't have their digestion working correctly. I have seen a greater number of clients correct their amazingly horrific symptoms and conditions by just correcting their digestion, more than any other issue. Like I talked about in chapter seven, one of our digestive processes is the acid that is formed in our stomach to help break down protein. But if you're not making enough acid, that meat doesn't get broken down. To understand how this is bad, try the following trick: Take a big bag of carrots and put them in a garbage can outside your house. Take another garbage can and fill it with raw meat. Let them sit there for about a week and go back, take the lid off and stick your head in each garbage can. Let me know which one smells worse. Which one did a better job of rotting, fermenting, attracting bugs and other crazy chemical reactions? If you don't want to do this experiment, I'll let you know: It's the meat.

So, just like in the trash can, if meat doesn't get properly digested, it will rot, ferment and create nasty chemicals that can throw off your body's balance and create issues, conditions and "disease."

But that doesn't mean that the real problem is the meat itself, it's just the fact that you can't break it down. Now that meat becomes something else—something else that you don't want in your body.

When Is Meat Healthy?

Does this help explain why so many authorities say that meat is bad for you? Why some vegetarians feel so much better when they stop eating meat? If their digestion isn't working well, they will feel much better "not digesting" vegetables than they did "not digesting" meat. Plus, if they were eating standard store- or restaurant-bought meat, they would feel better when they stopped putting all those drugs and chemicals into their systems. Nonetheless, this doesn't prove that meat is really bad for you. If you are a person who actually has your digestion working properly and you buy meat or eggs that come from organic, free-range animals, animal protein can be a very healthy part of your diet. With all the "studies" they do on eating meat and diseases that come from doing so, have you ever heard of a study using organic, free-range meats? It never happens. Have you ever heard of a study using only people with their digestion working properly? Of course not. 90% of the people with bad digestion don't even know that they have bad digestion.

The truth is, a lot of people really need animal protein. Here's how it works: Everything on the planet that eats, for the most part, is doing so to bring in nutrients and minerals so their body can function correctly. Well, these nutrients and minerals actually come from the Earth's soil. But as humans, we can't just pick up dirt and eat it because our body doesn't have the ability to process those nutrients. However, if we eat the plant that ate those minerals and nutrients from the soil (so to speak), we have an easier time translating those nutrients to something we can use in our bodies. If we take that a step further and eat the meat from the animal that ate that plant, the nutrients and minerals are even closer to a state that we can use.

273

Does this mean that you have to eat meat? Not necessarily. You can get a lot of the important nutrients you would get from meat by using the correct supplements. What it does mean is this: You don't have to stop eating meat to be healthy; and if you don't eat meat, you do need to supplement nutrients so you are getting the important nutrients that you're missing out on. But as long as your digestion is working correctly, the only thing left to do is buy good, quality meats and eggs that are organic, free-range and hormone-free. To the person with good digestion, everything is food; to the person with poor digestion, nothing is food. To quote my own book, "Diet is what a person eats but nutrition is what the cells see."

Vegan / Vegetarian

This is a fun section because I know everyone becomes defensive when they see the heading. "Is he going to make me just eat weeds?" or "Is he going to speak poorly of me and my vegan cohorts?" No matter what side of the fence someone stands on, most people simply don't want to hear about the other side. But you've figured out by now that I'm really not that nice and I'm probably going to end up bashing both sides, tear down the fence, and build a bonfire where we'll roast a pig and drink wheat grass juice, all at the same party.

First of all, I will say that I was vegan for nearly two years and it really is not as difficult as you may think. It's just a matter of creating new habits and learning new recipes. Everything else is just life and putting food choices into that life. (I don't know if that sentence makes any sense but I kinda like it for some reason.) If you have chosen to be a vegan or vegetarian because of your love for animals, or you hate the idea of eating anything with a face, or your religion tells you to "praise all creatures that can poop," or anything like that, then I suggest continuing that path. If that is what makes you happy, I won't argue with you. I, on the other hand, became a vegan because I thought that was the healthiest choice to make. Turns out... not so true.

When you first start eating vegetarian, you will often feel better, have better energy and you may lose weight as well. Let's look at why that happens. First of all, if you're eating the wrong kinds of meat or your digestion is not working well enough to break down the meat you were eating (as discussed under *What About Meat?* earlier in this chapter), then by eliminating that meat, you are taking away a burden that your body was dealing with while you were consuming meat. Now that your body doesn't have to deal with the chemicals, hormones and drugs that were in the meat, or your body doesn't have to try to digest a food that it doesn't have the resources to break down properly, now it can turn its attention to removing junk in the body. Anytime digestion is not working properly, vegetables will break down much easier than meat. By making the switch to a vegetarian diet, you also free up more resources, resulting in more energy. Vegetables also contain nutrients that will help bind to acids and other toxins, allowing them to be safely removed from the body, resulting in weight loss. Since you are now eating less meat, you will obviously be eating more vegetables so you will receive more of the benefits from these types of nutrients. Pretty good deal, huh? Well, that's not really the whole story.

Now pay attention because I'm about to sound smart. In the same way that vegetables contain nutrients that you need (nutrients you can't get from any other sources), so does animal protein. When you first stop eating meat, your body has a reserve of these nutrients that can be utilized for a period of time until you run out. Therefore, in the beginning, you're not overworking your digestive system by trying to eat meat that you can't digest, you're getting more good vegetable nutrients that your body needs in order to remove waste and toxins, and you still have a reserve of animal-based nutrients that your body can pull from as needed. It's all good, you feel great and you wonder why you didn't become a vegetarian a long time ago. As time passes, however, you begin to run out of the reserves of animal-based nutrients and you run into trouble. Your body will even begin to break down your own tissues to pull the nutrients required, as if you are the animal that your body is eating. As people begin to feel worse, they don't even consider the fact that they need animal protein because they felt so great in the beginning when they stopped eating it. Do you see how the confusion sets in?

Is eating vegetarian healthy for a lot of people? Sure. Especially if their digestion isn't working well enough to break down meat and the meat is just going to rot and ferment in their stomachs. But the truly optimal thing to do is to fix your digestion so you can actually break down the meat you eat, then, eat meat that is free of hormones, drugs and disease. Eating a diet that is far heavier in vegetables than meat is always the best plan. But I find that most people, at least in the long run, do need some form of meat (even if it's just eggs) in order to be fully healthy. If you are some type of ovo-vegetarian, or fresh water fish that begin with "t" vegetarian, or some new-fangled name that makes you feel more important than the rest of us, that may be a good route for you. Including some type of animal protein like fish, eggs, or chicken (even dairy can work well for many people), can be enough for a lot of people to get by on a vegetarian diet. If it isn't, you can always use supplements to try to fill in the missing pieces.

Vegetarianism And Weight Gain

Here's the real problem many vegetarians face: When you're eating less meat, you're eating less protein; and the protein you are eating is most commonly some type of processed vegetarian protein. So, if you are eating an ample amount of protein, it's probably a processed non-food that you are consuming. Also, when you eat less protein, that means you are likely eating more carbohydrates. More carbohydrates mean that you are going to spike your insulin levels higher. Higher insulin spikes send a signal to the body to store more fat and actually block your body's ability to burn fat for hours after the carbs have been burned. Yes, as a new vegetarian, you can begin to lose weight after the initial

276

release of toxins that were building up from undigested meat and chemicals you were consuming from eating the wrong meat. However, a lot of vegetarians have a hard time losing weight in the long run because they are eating so many complex carbohydrates that they block their body's ability to burn any stored fat as fuel.

Balance is always the best route.
Correcting digestion is always the first step.
It will always be that way.

Organic vs. Conventional

I'm going to share a couple viewpoints on this topic and one of them may surprise you. I've talked about how companies send me their products in hopes of winning one of our GearAwards on my site, www.ShapeYou.com. With this program, I really get to see a lot of new merchandise before it hits the market and I will say this: Nothing is more popular right now than slapping the word "organic" on a label. This is where the market is going. More people than ever are realizing the importance of buying organic. Since I like to hang out with the cool kids, let me first explain why buying organic is a good thing before I share the other viewpoint.

Wikipedia (which is always correct, right?) lists the definition of Organic Food as "foods that are produced using methods that do not involve modern synthetic inputs such as synthetic pesticides and chemical fertilizers, do not contain genetically modified organisms, and are not processed using irradiation, industrial solvents, or chemical food additives." If you combine this definition with what I wrote about chemicals and hormones found in meats, you can probably guess what I'm going to say next. When we eat foods that are filled with all these chemicals, where do you think those chemicals go? They go right into us, into our machines that we count on to carry us around all day. Just like any other synthetic or toxic substance that I've covered in this book, when these materials enter the body, the alarm sounds and the question is asked, "What the hell is this stuff?" When the human body encounters something that it doesn't recognize, it wants to send it out of the system. In essence, it becomes a problem to be dealt with.

People are starting to get the idea that if you're going to make the effort to eat healthier and swap out your corn chips for some broccoli, it might be a good idea to make sure the broccoli isn't loaded with harmful chemicals. Otherwise, you might as well stick with the corn chips.

Since the market is asking for organic products, organic products are starting to show up in places you might not expect to see them. It's fantastic that America's eyes are being opened to how harmful our despicable, almost bionic, farming methods have become. But it does freak me out a little to think about how some of the bigger corporations may take this organic foundation and start to figure out how to cut corners and save a buck. Until then, I will continue to enjoy the increased variety of organic foods available.

Fresh vs. Frozen

One thing that may surprise you is that frozen organic vegetables can sometimes be even better for you than the fresh produce. Most of the fresh produce you find in a store was picked days or even weeks ago and has been making its way through the handling process to show up on the shelf where you can buy it. During this time, the vegetable can cannibalize itself to stay alive. If you look at the bottom of a broccoli stem, you can often see where it has started to become hollow from the broccoli eating itself. Also, fresh produce is often picked before it is ripened so it can ripen during its travels. If the produce is picked early, its ability to absorb minerals was stunted by an early dismissal from the fields. Now this vegetable is not as dense with nutrients as it could have been if it matured properly.

Frozen vegetables are ripened on the vine and picked and frozen right away so all of that mineral stays intact. Plus, now you have the convenience of keeping vegetables in your freezer that are good for you.

Of course, the best way to go is to grow your own food or buy it at a trusted farmer's market where the produce was picked fresh. Not everyone has these options; but if you do, it's worth the extra effort or cost involved.

Organic Does Not Mean Healthy

I see this a lot. People will adapt to some new form of eating, whether it be vegan, organic, gluten-free, etc., and they think that as long as a food is gluten-free or organic, it must be healthy. Guess what? That's not even close to being true. If you make an organic candy bar, it's still a candy bar. Using organic ingredients doesn't change the fact that it's a pile of sugar that is going to spike your insulin levels. I will say that I do applaud the effort of some companies to remove chemicals, preservatives, artificial sweeteners and such, and make a sweet snack for kids that is sweetened by more natural things, like agave, honey or raw sugar. I applaud it, but that doesn't mean I would eat it or tell my clients to eat it. It is simply a step in the right direction. I appreciate the companies that are trying to provide an alternative to the submarine shaped non-food snack cakes that I grew up on. I have even been known to give a company an award for their attempts, even if it's a product I wouldn't eat myself. It's still something that is at least a 50% improvement over what else is out there, and I commend them on their efforts.

Organic just means that it doesn't include harmful chemicals. It's not a magic wand that automatically makes any food good for you. You still need to make good choices. Organic chocolate cake is still cake, and that sugar is going to pull calcium out of your tissues and increase your chances of having horrible cramps, despite its fancy organic label. Yes, by eating organic you can

279

eliminate some detrimental materials from entering your body, just do so intelligently. (I just had to use the spell corrector on the word "intelligently." Is that only funny to me?)

Organic Does Not Mean Nutritious

Here is the viewpoint that is often missed: Our food sucks. I mean, it contains a fraction of the nutrients that it did sixty years ago. Our "franken-farming" methods are making it possible for us to create beautiful looking produce that contains almost no minerals whatsoever. This is generally done by using chemicals that allow the plant to grow without the intended mineral, but this concern is not restricted to conventional farming methods by any means. Organic farming restrictions don't impose any rules on whether or not the soil needs to be properly replenished, or even contain appropriate amounts of mineral in the first place. This is where the mineral in our food comes from—the plant pulls it out of the soil. If the soil has been depleted, and proper methods have not been utilized to allow the earth to replenish itself, those organic crops are going to be missing nutrients.

You probably know that there are a variety of pests that can destroy farmers' crops. It is said that the mineral that exists within a plant is what helps the plant fight off pests that can destroy it. That is why conventional farming methods require pesticides—the lack of mineral in those crops has rendered them helpless to invaders. This is the basis of my optimism about organic farming. I like to believe that an organic crop must at least have enough mineral in it to survive without pesticides. I do not know that this is a fact, this is just an optimistic view that I hold on organic farming. However, my optimism does not mean that organic farmers are properly replenishing the soil, as they should. I agree that, when buying organic, we at least know that we are eliminating some poisons. It just doesn't mean that we're getting everything that is intended to be in that food. That organic food could still be lacking the nutrition that we are truly seeking. Studies have indicated that organic produce does contain more mineral than conventionally grown, but there is no way to show that this is true and consistent with all organic produce. The level of mineral within a food is more dependent on the soil it came from, rather than the organic label on the product itself.

Soil And Minerals

I want to dig deeper into this soil issue because I think it sheds some light on a lot of health issues that we're dealing with in America. (I just realized that I said, "dig deeper into the soil issue." I'm hoping you didn't think I was trying to be funny right there because that is weak.) It appears, as humans we are hard-wired for things that are sweet, because when food is the way it's supposed to be, where we find sweet is also where we find a lot of minerals. These minerals are what help us process the sugars in these sweet foods. That is why fruit is often not the healthy choice that it once was. The majority of fruit grown today is lacking the mineral needed to process the sugars contained in that fruit. The result can be a people thinking that they're making a healthy selection when they're really just eating a candy bar that grew on a tree.

To make matters worse, the industry will take a food like corn and process every single mineral out of it. First, they'll take out the germ and sell it for cattle feed. (Keep in mind, the germ is what "germinates." This is the life of the seed.) Next, they coat the remaining complex carbs with sugar to make it delicious and appealing to our senses. The brain sees this sweet product as having an abundance of mineral and says, "You need mineral badly, now eat a bucket of this stuff." An hour and a half after eating an entire bucket of sweet, nutritionally void "non-food," the person is looking for something else to eat. The body got ripped off and didn't receive what it thought it was getting, so it starts to look for something that can bring in the mineral that it needs.

The obesity problem in this country is not an issue of slackers who have no self-control at the dinner table. These are just people who are having their innate, hard-wired system used against them by the food manufacturers. Some of these food manufacturers make the people who make cigarettes look like upstanding citizens. At least they tell you right on the package that their product is not good for you. There are other factors often involved in obesity and you will be able to read about those in *Kick Your Fat in the Nuts*; but helping someone realize that they're not really eating food can be a big step in the right direction.

Beyond the processing of food, the real trouble with today's food source shows up when they begin to process the soil. People talk a lot about how the real problem is the American soil and how it has no mineral left in it. The Italians have been growing tomatoes for over 5,000 years, yet they still grow a good tomato. America has been farming for what, three hundred years? And we can't grow a tomato that tastes like anything anymore. You can see that it's red, but if you've ever talked to anyone who has eaten produce in other countries, they will tell you, "Over there, it actually has flavor in it." The American soil is not the problem, it is the American farmer. I've gone over how the mineral in the soil has to be there for that mineral to go into the plant. It's the bacteria in the soil, however, that allows the mineral to make that jump from the dirt to the plant, and into the fruit of that plant. The bacteria is the life of that soil. When you fertilize with these chemical and high phosphate fertilizers, you kill the bacteria and the mineral can't make the jump into the plant.

Nonetheless, for the first time in history, we now have brilliant scientists who have figured out how to engineer the seed so that it no longer requires these minerals to produce an apparent crop. Why do I say apparent? Because that's what the crops are: Produce that appears before you, even though it is void of mineral. Crops aren't even weighed anymore; they are sold by the bushel, which means they are sold by the size and not the weight. Mineral is what makes a crop weigh more, so there is no financial punishment for a farmer who sells a crop void of any significant food value. Are you following the path our food takes? We have the farmer "processing" the very soil and seed that our food comes from, then the product manufacturers "process" that produce into something that doesn't resemble food at all, and then we pray over it like the miracle of nature had anything to do with making it? Oops. That's why it's becoming so important to use good supplements that are appropriate for your body. This is becoming the only way to ensure that you're getting the nutrients you really need since our food supply is slowly turning into nothing more than something to chew on.

CHAPTER FIFTEEN (THE SUM UP)

Review & Make Your Plan

Now What?

I want to take a moment to lay out the important points that I've covered so you have an easy reference you can use to put your plan together. I know this was a lot of information and you may feel a little overwhelmed and excited at the same time. Just take a deep breath and I'll cover the important points that you don't want to forget and a few that will help you move forward and avoid some pitfalls.

You've learned an incredible amount of information so this section will be where I pull a Mr. Miyagi and help you put it all together in a usable format. By the end of this wrap-up, you should be saying, "Ah, that's why that bastard had me painting his fence."

Bring It All Together

Improving menstrual cramps is most commonly about moving the right resources to the correct locations. You want to make sure there is enough calcium at the tissue level to allow muscles to relax. In order to accomplish this, first make sure you are measuring your self-test numbers to guide your diet and supplement modifications. The next step is to make sure those measurements are not being pulled or skewed to the wrong places because you are consuming too many sugars or other carbohydrates.

Here are major points to remember:

1. Correct any digestive issues so you can pull needed resources out of the food you're eating. DON'T SKIP THIS.
2. Work toward correcting any imbalances that may be inhibiting those resources from being utilized in a proper manner.
3. If you showed an Electrolyte Deficiency Imbalance, increase mineral levels by adding unrefined salt (like sea salt), mineral drops, or other appropriate supplements.
4. Monitor your blood pressure. If your blood pressure is low, you still need to do more work to increase your mineral levels. Remember, blood pressure could be too high or too low. Measuring is like "looking before you leap."
5. Reduce any vitamin D that could be pulling calcium out of the tissues—especially if your urine pH is over 6.2 and you have cramps.
6. Reduce any sugar and complex carb intake. Sugars pull calcium out of the tissues just like vitamin D can. When combining sugars with carbohydrates, their effect on calcium leaving the tissues can be multiplied.
7. Use fatty acids properly, and only if you are not dealing with a Catabolic Imbalance. It's best to start using fatty acids just before your cramps would start and only use them in the morning. Fatty acids, like those found in salmon or in flax seed oil pearl capsules, can help push calcium back down to the tissue level. Since vegetable oils are fatty acids and America is over consuming vegetable oils, they need to be used judiciously.

These are some of the most important steps for women suffering from menstrual cramps. Since you have read this book, measured where your chemistry is, and understand how to monitor yourself, you know which of the above factors apply to you the most. Since everyone is different, some of the points may not be as important or even apply to you. Remember, this book was about figuring out your specific cause for menstrual cramps. It wasn't about reading a bunch of stuff and then just following the summary list at the end. It's about responding to measurements. You can't manage what you don't measure. Pay attention to where you are and make adjustments accordingly.

Fix Digestive Issues

By testing yourself, you know if you need to put some attention toward improving digestion. Odds are great that if you're reading this book, you do. Don't skip this step. You will not get the results you want if you don't improve digestion through supplementation. If you're not digesting food successfully, you have little chance of moving any resources to the right places. In order to get calcium and other minerals down to the tissue level, the minerals first need to exist in your body in high enough quantities. Pulling those minerals out of your food is a great way to accomplish that. Digestion is huge. Don't skip it.

Correct Your Imbalances

Taking steps toward correcting an imbalance and actually correcting an imbalance are not the same thing. For many symptom improvements to show up, you need to truly correct the imbalance that is causing those symptoms. If you take steps to correct an Electrolyte Deficiency Imbalance, but your blood pressure is still incredibly low and all your numbers are still pointing to an Electrolyte Deficiency Imbalance, then more needs to be done to correct the issue.

You don't want to be the girl who says, "I did what you told me to do and I still have cramps." Put more stock in your numbers than in what you are doing to correct them. If your self-test numbers still show an imbalance, the symptoms will often still be there to go right along with that imbalance. Just because you did some work to correct the imbalance doesn't mean that you did ENOUGH work to correct YOUR imbalance. For some, it will take more effort and more time to see the results and move the body closer to balance. If you are experiencing a stubborn imbalance, get help from a professional who can guide you. You're probably just missing a key point or doing some things to work against yourself as you try to create improvements.

Monitor Your Numbers

Monitoring is a crucial step. When a person starts feeling better, it becomes easy to forget why this improvement came to be. I see a lot of clients who do the work to see improvement and then they stop doing the right things, go back to their old habits, and wonder why their issues come back. You wouldn't work out for one month, lose some weight and expect that weight to continue to stay off if you stopped working out. You have to continue to be aware of how your body is operating if you want to continue to see results. Yes, the amount of work, or monitoring, you'll need to do may drastically decrease once the body is in balance. Monitoring less frequently will certainly be appropriate once you're feeling great. But you still need to check your numbers from time to time and make sure everything is going as planned. This will allow you to steer clear of many problems.

Don't Work Against Yourself

Taking steps in the right direction is absolutely the most important way to get started. However, the steps you take in the wrong direction still count. Continuing to eat a lot of sugar or starches is still going to pull calcium out of the tissues, even if you're adjusting other factors in your favor.

Don't forget that you now have the tools to correct the cravings that cause you to eat all that junk. By correcting those cravings, reducing starches and sugars becomes a lot easier.

Try to remember that there is already a lot working against you, and it is likely not your fault that you are dealing with these issues. I feel like the despicable farming methods used in this country have to be responsible for a lot of our deficiencies. You may feel people shouldn't have to work this hard at living, and you're right; but profiteering in the farming industry is a reality. Keep this in the back of your mind in case your issues return, so you can become vigilant again about taking the right steps. In the same way that it can be fun to grow a nice plant, it can also be enjoyable to continue feeling better and having more vitality.

Watch The Signs

Most women experience cramps only around their period. That doesn't mean you don't have other markers you can watch to get an idea of how you're progressing or increasing your vitality. If you can make needed adjustments before your period shows up, you won't have to wait until you're screaming at your toaster to know that you have not reached the level of improvement you had hoped for.

If you're experiencing things on this list, you know you have not likely made enough changes for long enough to greatly improve your cramps:

- Urine pH over 6.4
- Resting systolic blood pressure is less than 112
- Charley Horses
- Cold Sores or Fever Blisters
- Frequent Colds
- Depression
- Insomnia

- Cravings
- Muscle Twitches

Make Your Plan

If you fail to plan, you plan to fail. Is it a little annoying that I said that? Yes, it is. But if it gets you to put together a course of action, I'm okay with being annoying. It doesn't take much for life to get in the way. The good news is that every month you will have an unfriendly reminder that you have yet to take the time to make the needed improvements. Writing up a plan in a notebook can help you avoid that reminder.

Since what you eat counts, know what you're going to eat before it's time to eat. If you wait until you're starving to decide what you're going to eat that day, you're going to end up with a scoop of Golden Grahams in a taco shell. Once major hunger strikes, all proper judgment can go out the window. Plan what you're going to eat ahead of time and you will make better choices.

In a similar vein, grocery stores have a magic threshold that erases your brain as you walk in the sliding glass doors. Know what you're going to buy before you get there.

If you find that you need to use supplements to improve digestion or an imbalance, plan that as well. Most of us live our lives on the go. Burger King doesn't carry the supplements you need, so you can't just drive through and grab them while you're out. Success will take making some new habits, but if you plan ahead, everything gets easier.

You're not going to just make one plan and stick with that forever. Remember that your plan will be adjusted as the measurements change on your *Data Tracking Sheet*.

Avoid Screwing Yourself Over

There really is no such thing as a "side effect"—only direct effects. When you use a supplement or change your diet, or increase or decrease water intake... all these things have the ability to change your body chemistry, and that change can create an effect. It's not a side effect; you did something and things changed. It's a direct effect.

I have heard "side effect" described as choosing to put up with poisonous or negative effects in order to have a particular benefit. Don't you think the better choice is to have only benefit? Let's choose the positive without the price of a negative.

Avoid looking at these changes like, "This doesn't work for me," and therefore quit trying to balance your body. Whatever change you are creating is just more information. If something creates the opposite reaction than what you're looking for, then you can use that information to steer in the right direction. If you understand how to look at the clues, you don't have to jump ship just because a bird crapped on the deck of the boat.

If you choose a course of action, and your measurements show things going in the opposite direction, try to remember a change in measurement that goes in the opposite direction is still wonderful information. You're finding your way. If a supplement or food choice doesn't work, that information can go a long way in determining what WILL work for you. Why did a choice push you in the opposite direction? Use that information to look for an answer. Find a practitioner to help you decipher why anything might push you in the wrong direction.

Here are two examples. A young lady by the name of Soupy was having stomach pains. (Good thing I changed her name for this book. That would have been very unfortunate if her name was really Soupy.) Soupy's body was not creating enough stomach acid to break down the food she was eating. As her food would rot and ferment, gases were created that would expand her intestines and cause pain and bloating. She started using HCL supplements and immediately her pain began to reduce. But she also started experiencing painful heartburn.

Remember that the LES valve at the bottom of the esophagus is triggered to close when stomach acid levels rise due to digestion kicking in. Without enough stomach acid, that valve doesn't close and you can have reflux. If there is no stomach acid, you won't even feel that reflux because there is no acid coming up to burn you. If you begin to add HCL supplementation, now you have some acid in your stomach. But if you haven't reached a high enough dose to trigger that valve to close, now you have reflux that contains acid and you get burned. This can happen even if you are avoiding carbohydrates while you initially begin increasing HCL intake (as explained in chapter twelve.)

Soupy thought that since she had never experienced heartburn before, it must be the HCL that was giving her heartburn so she stopped using it. If she would have just increased her dosage according to instructions, her acid levels would have triggered the valve to close, reflux would stop and she could have continued receiving the relief from her stomach pains that follow every meal for her. By misunderstanding what her body was telling her, she eliminated an opportunity to improve her health and eliminate a horrible discomfort she lives with every day.

Another example is what happened to Sugarplum. Yes, her name really is Sugarplum. Sugarplum wanted to correct her Electrolyte Deficiency Imbalance and also lose weight. She began using supplements to improve her imbalance and correct her digestion. She lowered her carb intake so her insulin would not spike as often and cause her body to store fat. This helped her to drop weight.

But her cravings for sugar also began to skyrocket. She had never had uncontrollable cravings before so she assumed that the supplements she was using had messed up her body in some way and caused her to be a sugar freak so she stopped taking supplements. This is a fun deduction, but as an option, we could also use science and logic to figure out what happened to Sugarplum.

You learned earlier that cravings are mostly created from low minerals and/or low blood sugar. Sugarplum was taking the right steps to improve her Electrolyte Deficiency Imbalance but her imbalance was strong and her blood pressure was still extremely low, indicating that she still had a low level of minerals in her system. Once she lowered her carb and sugar intake to lose weight, there was now nothing left to buffer the system—not enough minerals and not enough sugars. Cravings almost always skyrocket when sugars and minerals are both low.

Before she started attempting to raise her mineral levels with supplements, she never had cravings because she was buffering her system with carbs and sugars (which is the reason she had gained weight in the first place). As long as sugars are high, a person won't get those cravings. Weight gain often shows up as a result of keeping those sugars high, but the uncontrollable cravings can be kept at bay.

If Sugarplum would have added some medium carb foods (not starch) to her diet, instead of eliminating all carbs, the sugars from those carbs could have continued to buffer her low mineral content. Her weight loss would have been more gradual, but that's okay since she would also be keeping her cravings away. As her mineral content and blood pressure began to climb, she could have reduced her carbs further at that point if she still needed to lose weight. The important lesson here is not to look at the changes you make as "not working" or "causing crazy side effects." As we discussed, these were all direct effects—not side effects. These effects just needed to be looked at logically so she could use them to steer her next move.

The moral of both these examples is this: Don't screw yourself. Most people never have an opportunity to correct the issues that are plaguing them. Don't screw yourself out of that opportunity because you decide to ignore how your system works. Listen to the clues that show up. If they don't make sense to you, get help from someone who can help you decipher them. Stay determined and keep in mind why you started this journey. You can kick your menstrual cramps in the nuts if you're willing to just do the work. Do a self-test. Measure your numbers so your situation will make sense to you. Then, you can regulate what is needed.

Finding Supplements

Remember, a lot of the supplements I talk about in this book will not be found in stores. Most products that I talk about in this book can be found on NaturalReference.com. Don't forget about digestion when ordering supplements. If you're like most of the readers of this book, digestion will be the priority and you will likely be ordering Betaine HCL, Beet Flow, and Omnizyme to cover all three aspects of digestion. All three of these products are available without a health coach.

Continue To Learn

Just like anything, the more you learn, the easier it becomes not to suck at it. Continue learning. Visit our website at www.KickItInTheNuts.com and soak in piles of free information. Use the code "skedaddle" to register for free as a veteran book reader so you can access all the good stuff.

Hidden Chapter

Earlier in this book, I mentioned a "Hidden Chapter" that I placed on my website, www.KickItInTheNuts.com. I've set it up so you can read this chapter and send it to a friends. It can be a good way to introduce your friends to the world of "understanding your own body."

Also, feel free to drop me a line. I'd love to get any feedback, even if that feedback includes cussing. I just like to get mail. I won't be able to answer any questions about your specific chemistry or health issues because there are piles of laws that prohibit that if you're not a personal client of mine. But if you just bought some ninja socks at the store and want to tell me about it, I'd love to hear from you.

Ask F'in Tony & The Community Forum

Even though I'm not allowed to answer questions about your specific chemistry, I've still set you up to get the answers you need. Go to www.KickItInTheNuts.com and register for free so you can interact with other readers as well as the guy who wrote this (me). Click on "Ask F'in Tony" to submit a general question to me directly. If I select your question, I'll post the answer so the whole community can learn. You can also search through previous answers to see if I have already covered a topic you are trying to figure out.

If I don't select your question to be featured in my "Ask F'in Tony" section, you can always browse the community forum. Here you can share information with other readers, or even ask questions to see if anyone might have an answer that could be helpful.

Book Updates

My co-authors and I are constantly learning more about nutrition and how the body really works. Once you register on www.KickItInTheNuts.com with the book reader code "skedaddle," be sure to click on BOOK TOOLS > BOOK UPDATES, and find this book title to read about any findings we have come across since we released this book.

Follow Me

You can find my social fanciness at:

www.facebook.com/KickItInTheNuts
www.twitter.com/KickItInTheNuts

My First Movie

If you're not sick of me yet, go to the site for my documentary, *Why Am I So Fat?*. You can watch trailers and videos, and by the time you read this book, the movie may be out.

www.WhyAmISoFatMovie.com
www.facebook.com/FatMovie
www.twitter .com/SoFatMovie

Your Top Secret Book Reader Code

skedaddle

Be Excited

Right now, in your hand, you are holding answers that some people search for their entire lives and never find. You now have knowledge that can be the "cheat sheet" to your health and your life. Don't take it for granted.

Final Words

For the final words of this book, I select wheelbarrow and horse collar.

APPENDIX A

11-Parameter Urine Dipstick
&
Advanced Testing Details

11-Parameter Urine Dipstick

On the website, www.NaturalReference.com, you can find a product, Urispec 11-way urine test strips. A canister of 100 test strips will run you about $45 and very few people will need to order these more than once. These strips are an excellent tool to give you insights that you would normally learn only by visiting a health professional. The Urispec 11-way urine test strips (also referred to as a 10-parameter urine test strip) measure blood, urobilinogen, bilirubin, protein, nitrite, ketones, ascorbic acid, glucose, pH, specific gravity and leukocytes. Not only can these measurements help you recognize which imbalances may be the most severe for you, but also, individuals could uncover some fairly major issues that could cause all kinds of trouble if undetected. In my opinion, with these test strips, people can uncover information that may be more valuable to their health than anything they would find in most traditional blood tests—all for about forty five cents a strip.

When using an 11-parameter urine test strip, all of the measurements can be read right away except the leukocytes reading. You want to start a two-minute egg timer as soon as you dampen the test strip and read the leukocytes box right at that two-minute time. Pee into a cup and then dip the strip all the way into the cup. You may have to bend the strip a little by pushing the strip against the bottom of the cup in order to get all the colored boxes covered in urine. Pull the strip out right away and tap its edge on a paper towel to wick away some of the excess urine. Read the colors against the color chart on the strips container. On the *Data Tracking Sheet*, circle the colored boxes that match the colors on your dipstick for each reading.

I'll talk about each independent variable on this dipstick later in this appendix when I cover Advanced Tests. But this dipstick is a great, cheap way to look at some more in-depth numbers. I recommend using this 11-parameter dipstick at least once to get a bigger picture of what is going on with your body.

Below, I give you details that help explain what you're looking at when you view each of the parameters on this dipstick. Some of the words are all big and fancy. You don't really need to understand them right now. I just want to let you know what's available on these dipsticks.

Non-Hemolyzed / Hemolyzed

Non-Hemolyzed indicates parts of red blood cells dropping into the urine. Hemolyzed blood does not drop into the urine. Blood is not something you want to see in your urine. Blood in the urine would certainly be an indication of either kidney or bladder distress or trauma. Sometimes non-hemolyzed blood seen during an individual's monthly cycle would not be regarded as significant until a test outside that time of month confirms the indication.

Bilirubin

Bilirubin should be going out the biliary pathway, it should not be seen in the blood or urine. Bilirubin is processed from biliverdin. The spleen is pulling out the old blood cells, the biliverdin is sent over to the liver, the liver then changes the biliverdin into

297

bilirubin, and bilirubin is going into the bile. When bilirubin is seen in the urine, that means that it did not go out the biliary pathway, down through the intestines and out the south gate (your butt). It is a validator that the biliary pathway isn't running as nicely as it should. Since bile flow is so important for digestion and waste removal, this is an excellent parameter to have access to.

Urobilinogen

Urobilinogen is bilirubin that has been eaten for lunch in the intestines by bacteria. When they eat bilirubin, they poop urobilinogen. This can be common if an individual is constipated. Since the stool is moving at a much slower pace, it allows this bacteria to thrive.

Protein

Protein should not be seen in the urine. If it is, that can be an indicator that the kidneys may be overwhelmed. Protein in the urine can also be an indicator that the body is breaking down its own tissue.

Nitrite

Nitrite is a byproduct produced by bacteria. If the dipstick reads positive in any way then it is one of the indicators that there is a UTI (urinary tract infection)—some type of bacteria in the bladder.

Ketones

Ketones are produced by the burning of fat. Typically diabetics show ketones because they are not burning carbohydrates, they are burning fat. People on the Atkins Diet were given ketone strips to show that they had reached the goal of ketosis, so that they would burn fat. This switch to burning fat didn't seem to harm anyone to speak of because the body can function that way.

Even hypoglycemic people will also show ketosis if they haven't eaten for some time before the testing.

Ascorbic Acid (A Fractionated form of Vitamin C)

Ascorbic acid will alter the readings on the dipstick. So while this reading lets you know how much ascorbic acid might be being excreted in the urine, it also alerts you that some of the reagents may react improperly when there is too much ascorbic acid.

Glucose

The dipstick color chart shows that some glucose in the urine is "normal." I might agree that is "common" however one would not want to conclude that it is optimal or "normal." I don't think it is correct that glucose should be in people's urine. Typically you see a glucose reading in the negative box, showing no glucose—that is how you want to see it. If you do see glucose in the urine, in connection with nitrite and leukocytes on the dipstick, now you know what the bacteria in the bladder are munching on. They are munching on glucose in the urine. The bacteria are hopped up on sugar and having a party.

pH

Because many people are already measuring pH with instruments, pH from the dipstick standpoint is a validator that you have calibrated your instruments correctly. If it doesn't read the same as your instruments, then somebody is wrong. It is not a high-fidelity test of pH, but if you're using any other equipment or any other type of pH strip, it's a nice validation.

Specific Gravity

Specific gravity can be used to validate whether or not your body is leaning too anabolic or too catabolic. This alone is not an indication, however, it can be a great piece of data when looking for further confirmation.

Measuring on a dipstick is not a high-fidelity test of specific gravity because it is only measuring ionized dissolved solids. Using equipment to measure specific gravity will bring a more accurate reading, but this is a convenient way to find a range.

Leukocytes

This reading shows leukocytes coming from the bladder, not necessarily from the whole system. Leukocytes are joined right away to nitrite; and if you see them both in the urine, that is a very positive indicator of a urinary tract infection and bacteria in the bladder. If you see one of them then you would certainly be wondering if that is a situation that this individual is having trouble with, but it is not as positive as seeing both of them.

Advanced Tests

Here I explain some advanced tests I haven't covered, but I also go over other tests that I talked about in chapter four. I want to cover them again here so I can give you additional information. I showed you how to look at some of these measurements using strips and other simple tools, but you can also measure some of these parameters using equipment, so placing them in this advanced section is a good fit. I cover the familiar tests first.

Tests You Can Do Now

pH of Urine and Saliva

pH is like looking at barometric pressure. Which way are things going? pH of urine and pH of saliva give you a view of the potential direction the system is leaning. Urine is the trash can of life, that's what you're throwing out. Saliva is what you're holding on to. It can't be said that saliva is interstitial fluid, but it can give you a clue of what the fluid is like between the cells (otherwise known as the intercellular fluid). When you compare what is being thrown out against what's being held onto by the saliva, you can start to get some discernment about what's going on. That's how you begin to get a picture of how your body is operating. These readings can be very enlightening because neither urine nor saliva are compensated fluids like the blood.

Resting Blood Pressure and Standing Blood Pressure

Resting blood pressure lets you know how well the system is working overall. The blood pressure, along with the pulse, can be a nice overview of what type of resources the system has at its disposal, and even whether or not junk is being properly removed. When a person stands, the system is stressed a slight bit. The response to that stress then gives indications as to how panicked the system is. If you can't stand up with relative ease, and without the system going into what would be interpreted as an overreaction, then your system is likely not doing well.

Pulse

The optimum resting pulse count for an adult is in the range of 68 to 77 beats per minute. Pulse rate is an indicator of the body's ability to adapt to its environment. Can it adapt easily, with a slightly elevated pulse rate? Does the need to adapt cause a desperate response that can alter other systems in a negative way? A pulse that is too rapid is showing the system in distress. A pulse that is too slow is also providing useful information—not necessarily an indication of being very fit, as is often believed. The pulse rate can be slow or fast due to many variables, including: blood viscosity, thick or thin; a fever, the immune system on high alert; acid-tending or alkaline-tending blood.

Breath Rate and Breath Hold are the most reliable measurements to identify if your blood is leaning too alkaline or too acid. They are indicating the pH of the bloodstream and how easily the kidneys are maintaining control of that parameter. If the breath rate is fast and the breath hold is short, one would conclude the bloodstream is tending to drift to the acid side. If the breath rate is slow and the breath hold is long, it could be concluded that the bloodstream is tending toward the alkaline side. Going either way starts to compromise or diminish oxygen transportation by the bloodstream. This lowered oxygen transport can alter the way energy has to be produced in the body.

Blood Glucose

A blood glucose reading that is out of range is an excellent indicator that there is high insulin in the system. However, if blood glucose is in range, it doesn't mean that the pancreas isn't producing a lot more insulin than it should have to. Blood glucose isn't the ideal measurement. I wish there was a method to easily measure insulin, too. You see, glucose can be in a normal range, say 80-90; but behind the curtain, the body is cranking out tons of insulin in order to keep the glucose in that range. If this goes on too long, the cells will become resistant to the insulin and the body can stop processing insulin all together. Then the blood glucose levels will sky rocket, as if from nowhere. Although looking at this parameter can let you know you're in big trouble if glucose numbers are very high, having a glucose reading that is in range does not necessarily mean that everything is running smoothly. Wow, I think that just helped me understand that rule stating that a square is always a rectangle but a rectangle isn't always a square. I just nodded when they said that but had no idea what my teachers were talking about.

Body Temperature

Everyone knows that a high temperature is a fever and it is generally accepted that a fever isn't necessarily a bad thing. The hypothalamus resets the body to a higher temperature to make the system less hospitable to an invader. If the temperature is high, you start trying to figure out how to assist the body in its effort to make things very uncomfortable for the invader. On the same token, a low temperature is indicating that there is a problem with energy production. Enzymes don't fire right if the body temperature is too low; so if a person has a low body temperature, we can also look for other signs of digestive issues.

Dermographic Line

This is an autonomic nervous system indicator. Typically if a person's vascular system is constricted, the dermographic line stays with a white center and can indicate the individual is leaning too far on the sympathetic side. If the dermographic line stays red, that can indicate a person is leaning towards the parasympathetic side. Sympathetic is the "Fight or Flight" state. "Rest and Digest" is the parasympathetic side. But again, it's not that the sympathetic side is right or wrong, or the parasympathetic side is right or wrong. They are both correct and appropriate in certain circumstances. Can the body adapt? Does the body have the ability to choose either side? Or has some type of higher priority, such as electrolytes, become so whacked that now the balance of the autonomic nervous system is no longer a choice?

Look at it this way: Imagine you were having a bad hair day and your attention was on trying to avoid having "Diana Ross head." But your hand slipped and now your curling iron is stuck to your ear and it's making a sizzling noise and it's apparent you will be passing out soon from the pain. Because the higher priority of horrible pain has taken precedence, you've forgotten about your hair and that issue is now put on the back burner (I didn't mean to

303

use a burner analogy while your ear was is still sizzling). At least this illustrates how an imbalance can sometimes exist in the body merely because priorities have been shifted to other areas.

Gag Reflex

Gag reflex is another indicator of the autonomic nervous system. High gag reflex is indicating that a person is leaning towards the parasympathetic side. The lack of a gag reflex indicates a leaning toward the sympathetic side. No test is required here. Simply ask yourself, if I'm brushing my teeth and the toothbrush goes a little too far back, do I gag?

Pupil Size

Pupil size is another indicator of the autonomic nervous system. Small pupils indicate parasympathetic; large pupils indicate sympathetic. Looking at the colored area of your eye, if your pupils cover less than 25% of that space, they can be considered small. If your pupils cover more than 50% of the colored area, they can be considered large. If your pupils take up between 25% - 50% of the colored space, this can be considered normal.

Tests That Need Advanced Equipment And Education

Conductivity / Millisiemens (mS) of Urine and Saliva

This demonstrates the electrical conductivity of the urine and saliva. The speed at which an electrical current will flow through those two fluids can indicate many things—kidney function and digestive capacity, for example. It can even be an indication of how the liver is functioning because the kidneys may become overburdened very quickly if the liver isn't operating correctly. Viewing mS along with urine pH and saliva pH is a better way to get an idea of how the liver is functioning. Conductivity and millisiemens are the same thing. Millisiemens and conductivity are different scales for the same measurement, just as meters and yards are measuring length, using different markings. One side of the measuring stick uses the metric system and the other side of the measuring stick uses the imperial system, because people get comfortable with different measurement systems.

rH2 of Urine and Saliva

rH2 is closely related to pH, but pH is looking only at hydrogen. rH2 is looking at all the other ions in the system and their electrical charge. That electrical charge indicates how hard the atmosphere is pushing in a certain direction. Digestion is a huge topic, and HCL is crucial to digestion. rH2 can give us some big clues as to whether or not the body is producing HCL. It's not an "HCL meter" so to speak, but it can give outstanding clues in that direction.

Surface Tension of Urine

Surface tension of urine is letting you see how many byproducts from energy production are being poured out in the urine. Since the surface active components of energy production through oxidation tend to lower surface tension, whether energy is being produced through oxidation or fermentation can be seen from the surface tension measurement when put in a context of other parameters such as pH and even the time of day the measurement is taken. Yeah, that's a heap of science right there. Of course, you need to know what I'm talking about for this to make sense. But at least you know this piece of information can help a professional health coach understand how your body is processing the foods you eat.

Specific Gravity of Urine and Saliva

Specific gravity is the amount of dissolved solids in that solution. When sugar or salt break down in water, these are solids that have dissolved. Specific gravity is the amount of dissolved solids in a solution. There is a point when a solution is no longer able to break down a solid and it will be held in suspension for as long as the solution is being stirred. When the stirring stops, the solid falls. It is no longer in suspension but has "salted out" and is at the bottom of the glass. Those that stay up in the solution are dissolved solids. Specific gravity can give some indications as to whether or not a person is dealing with an anabolic or catabolic imbalance.

NO3 and NH4 of Urine and Saliva (and the information we can pull from the relationship between the two)

These measurements are giving you clues and indications as to what is happening with protein. Dr. Reams mentioned that the NO3 of urine is letting you see inbound protein and the NH4 of urine is letting you see the outbound protein. NO3 of saliva is looking specifically at bacterial activity in the mouth only; it is not looking at a system-wide issue. If this number goes high, like over 14, it can be an indication of a high amount of bacteria waste in the mouth. It's not very pleasant to think about bacteria pooping in your mouth all day long; yet it can be a reality for those who have poorly executed dental work which may have left holes or pockets in the gums where bacteria can flourish.

The majority of NH4 is produced in the kidneys, and allows other testing numbers to gain greater credibility when they are reviewed with NH4.

Vitamin C Test

Vitamin C is really the superglue that is holding the human body together. Vitamin C is used in nearly every repair process in the body. Humans, guinea pigs and primates are the only mammals that don't make their own Vitamin C. With this in mind, it's very important that all of us get enough Vitamin C from our food or through supplementation. The Vitamin C test can give you an indication of what is going on with Vitamin C in the system.

Learn More

To learn more about advanced testing equipment or where you can take courses teaching how to use these advanced testing methods, contact us at www.KickItInTheNuts.com

APPENDIX B

Those Who Paved the Way

Dr. Carey Reams

Dr. Carey Reams was an agrarian. He did soil chemistry and he learned, primarily, how to make things grow in the soil. By people coming to him for help, he was pushed into biology and working with animals and humans. What remained at the root of his mentality was all this knowledge about what made produce grow exceptionally well. What needed to be done in order to bring the proper level of minerals into the produce? What got a result in the crop? There are a lot of stories about how Reams adjusted minerals in the soil to affect the growth of produce. If you wanted to do something in soil, he knew how to do it. That mentality was then brought forward into looking at health from a simple ground-up standpoint. Reams looked at the mineral content in a person, much like he looked at the mineral content in the soil.

Dr. Emanuel Revici

Dr. Emanuel Revici was all about looking at the cell's oil-based membrane and the proteins that are mixed in with it. He explained what was going on with the permeability of the cells. Through learning about cellular permeability, we came to understand that there is a natural tide to life, or a rhythm. This is where the anabolic/catabolic language comes into use. We see that during the daytime it is proper for a person to be in a catabolic state—when he is giving his energy to the day. Conversely, as surely as night falls and the dandelion flower closes, the anabolic state is entered and the person goes to sleep to rebuild and restore himself. Everyone needs to be cycling between these two states. As people lose their vitality or resilience, this tide of life becomes impeded and an individual can get stuck in the anabolic or catabolic state 24 hours a day.

Without the necessary vitality to allow this natural oscillation process to continue, it is statistically true that those who become stuck in an anabolic state are more prone to viral issues occurring in their system. Those who have lost their resilience and are stuck in a catabolic state are more prone to bacterial issues. Now comes the reasonableness of the system where if a person is really oscillating every evening from catabolic to anabolic, and every morning from anabolic going back to catabolic, then the viruses don't have a home and the bacteria don't have a home because the system is oscillating. There is never a moment when, for many many days, there is a hospitable environment for those issues to take hold.

There is a good book about Dr. Revici, written by William Kelley Eidem, called *The Doctor Who Cures Cancer*. This is a story of Revici's life and work and is an excellent introduction into the intellect he provided us.

Thomas Riddick

Thomas Riddick understood colloidal suspensions. What is the bloodstream? It is a colloidal suspension. This is information that painters understand perfectly because, if you can't keep pigment in suspension, then it is going to separate, fall to the bottom of the can and harden. If that pigment falls out of suspension then you aren't going to sell much paint. You aren't going to get the pigment to the wall, it's not going to dry correctly and it isn't going to work. With Riddick's research, we came to understand a lot more about the heart and how to make the bloodstream flow easier so that the heart does not work so hard.

Certainly, when half of America is dying from a heart-related problem, we would be curious to know what to do to make things easier for the heart. That used to be understood before profit-driven thinking took over. I don't want that to sound like I'm bitter, I'm not. I do wish that those who put profit over the public's well-being could be locked in a room and forced to listen to old Menudo albums until they promise to change their ways, but I'm not bitter. I don't want you to think that I'm the type of person that would basically Menudo-style waterboard someone. Still, wouldn't the world be a better place? If this was taken care of, the only issues we would need to get rid of are smoking in public, people who stink, and those that drive slow in the left lane. Order restored.

Dr. Melvin Page

Dr. Melvin Page was a dentist whose research showed that proper nutritional balance in the body could not only improve the health of someone's teeth, but also the health of the body would coincide with the improvement of their dental health. He found that, when the calcium-to-phosphorus ratio was in a balanced proportion, the patient would present no cavities. (The actual proportion is ten-to-four in the blood, for those who like it when I say things that make me sound fancy. For those who say, "What the hell is he talking about?" just use the word "balanced.") Moving outside of this ratio would not only present cavities, but other health issues as well.

Dr. Page was also very interested in, and had a lot of success with, hormones. He found that you couldn't even get a good read on hormones if the blood sugar was elevated. For this reason, he would require avoidance of carbohydrates for at least 72 hours before any hormone testing was done. When we look around us today, with the rate that the population is having trouble with diabetes, hypoglycemia, and blood sugar issues, is it any wonder that there are also a lot of hormonal issues going on? Dr. Page had a lot of information that we try to implement.

Dr. Page and all these other doctors serve to validate or challenge each other's views. It's as though they're all looking into the same room (human physiology) but through different windows, giving a different perspective on very similar issues.

Recommended Reading

The Doctor Who Cures Cancer - William Kelley Eidem
> The story of Emanuel Revici, M.D. that introduced us to the anabolic/catabolic shifts in the body.

Nutrition and Your Mind - George Watson
> An excellent book that demonstrates how the types of foods we eat can make a difference in our physical health and mental health.

More About Tony

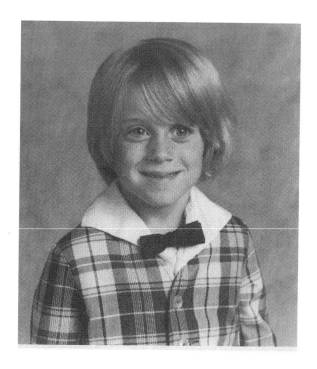

Like most natural health experts, Tony began his career in stand-up comedy. Touring professionally as a comic for nearly a decade, he never envisioned that he would one day teach the world how to sleep, poop, and even lose weight.

On Valentine's Day, 2004, Tony lost his voice and it never came back. After twenty-three doctors couldn't figure out the problem, Tony decided it was time to dig for his own answers. Eight years later, not only did Tony figure out his own issues, he also happened upon hidden information about how to improve countless other health problems.

Though Tony likes to boast about the fact that he holds no legitimate credentials (nor does he believe that we need any more "experts" from the same pool of knowledge already failing so many with health issues), he is greatly respected by his peers in the natural health industry. The biggest manufacturers in the health, fitness and organic products industries send Tony their products every year in hopes of winning one of his GearAwards.

Beyond working with many celebrity clients, Tony is on the executive board of the *Coalition for Health Education*, a nonprofit association that helps professionals and their clients learn about health through nutrition. Additionally, Tony teaches monthly webinars about nutrition to doctors, nutritionists and other health care professionals from more than thirty-five countries.

You can also find Tony producing documentaries like, *Why Am I So Fat?* A film that teaches the truth about weight loss while showcasing Tony's client, Gabe Evans, who lost 200 pounds in 9 ½ months by treating Tony's word as gospel.

To learn more about Tony, visit www.KickItInTheNuts.com

That's it. Close the book now.

Proof

Made in the USA
Charleston, SC
29 May 2012